CARDIO
ESSENTIALS

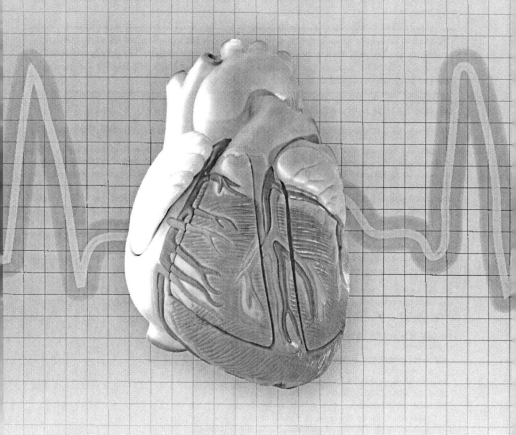

TERESA HOLLER, MS, PA-C

Cardiology Physician Assistant
Consultants in Cardiology
Roanoke, Virginia

JONES AND BARTLETT PUBLISHERS
Sudbury, Massachusetts
BOSTON   TORONTO   LONDON   SINGAPORE

World Headquarters

Jones and Bartlett Publishers	Jones and Bartlett Publishers	Jones and Bartlett Publishers
40 Tall Pine Drive	Canada	International
Sudbury, MA 01776	6339 Ormindale Way	Barb House, Barb Mews
978-443-5000	Mississauga, Ontario L5V 1J2	London W6 7PA
info@jbpub.com	CANADA	UK
www.jbpub.com		

Jones and Bartlett's books and products are available through most bookstores and online booksellers. To contact Jones and Bartlett Publishers directly, call 800-832-0034, fax 978-443-8000, or visit our website www.jbpub.com.

Substantial discounts on bulk quantities of Jones and Bartlett's publications are available to corporations, professional associations, and other qualified organizations. For details and specific discount information, contact the special sales department at Jones and Bartlett via the above contact information or send an email to specialsales@jbpub.com.

Library of Congress Cataloging-in-Publication Data
Holler, Teresa.
  Cardiology essentials / Teresa Holler.
     p. ; cm.
  Includes bibliographical references and index.
  ISBN-13: 978-0-7637-5076-3
  ISBN-10: 0-7637-5076-X
  1. Cardiology. 2. Heart--Diseases. 3. Cardiovascular
system--Diseases. 4. Physicians' assistants. 5. Nurse practitioners.
I. Title.
  [DNLM: 1. Heart Diseases--diagnosis. 2. Heart Diseases--therapy. 3.
Nurse Practitioners. 4. Physician Assistants. WG 141 H7372c 2008]
  RC667.H65 2008
  616.1--dc22
                              2007006289
6048

Production Credits

Executive Editor: David Cella	Manufacturing and Inventory Coordinator:
Editorial Assistant: Lisa Gordon	Amy Bacus
Production Director: Amy Rose	Composition: Spoke & Wheel/Jason Miranda
Production Editor: Daniel Stone	Cover Design: Kristin E. Ohlin
Associate Marketing Manager: Jen Bengtson	Printing and Binding: Malloy, Inc.
	Cover Printing: Malloy, Inc.

Printed in the United States of America
11 10 09 08 07   10 9 8 7 6 5 4 3 2 1

Contents

Section IV: Cardio Conditions   145

Section V: Devices   235

Section VI: Lifestyles   249

Section VII: Survival Skills   259

Section VIII: Appendices   265

Preface

After a decade of precepting physician assistant (PA), nurse practitioner (NP), and medical students during the clinical portion of their training, I began teaching PA students during their didactic year. I noticed a troublesome void in cardiology books geared specifically toward PAs/NPs.

The perfect cardiology book for PAs and NPs should be enjoyable to read, easy to understand, evidence based, and exceedingly practical. Difficult cardiac concepts should be explained in a simplistic manner. Both those in primary care and specialty fields should be able to read the entire book in several nights and feel more comfortable treating cardiac patients.

Cardiology Essentials is the culmination of these goals. It is not a comprehensive review of heart disease, which would dilute the pearls and practical suggestions offered within. Instead, it is a handbook of practical advice from a seasoned cardiology PA and former assistant professor on how to become an efficient, competent part of the cardiology team. To accomplish this, *Cardiology Essentials* focuses primarily on the topics that are most relevant to PAs and NPs.

Cardiology Essentials is perfect for a broad audience because it offers text pieces called *Back to the Basics*, which teach basic concepts to beginners. More advanced information for the seasoned practitioner is also presented. Experienced providers may wish to skip the *Back to the Basics* sections and move to the more advanced material. Beginners may wish to omit the more advanced concepts until later in their course of study.

To keep the material light and easy to read, *Cardiology Essentials* incorporates many personal anecdotes to both entertain and educate the reader. Sidebars include *Bottom Line*, which summarize important information concisely throughout the text and *Pearls*, which provide clinically useful information gathered through years of experience. These personal paradigms and sidebars result in a product that is unique to medical education. It is actually pleasant to read! The book accomplishes this by also using the most recent clinical guidelines and evidence-based medicine. This approach has created a practical, clinically relevant book that can be read from cover to cover with ease.

The chapters in *Cardiology Essentials* cover such basics as *cardiac H&P*, with tips for constructing a comprehensive cardiac H&P; *ECG tricks* reveals quick tricks for assessing the ECG for clinically relevant information. The *Stress-free Stress Testing and Other Cardiac Studies* chapter explains various diagnostic studies and provides the PA/NP with the information they need to perform stress tests and tilt table studies. Section II, covering *Cardio Med*, reviews both basic and advanced details about cardiac drugs. The *Cardio Consults* section addresses some of the most common reasons the PA/NP is asked to see a patient and how to handle these consultations. The following information on *Cardio Conditions* provides the most recent clinical guidelines on the most common conditions that PAs and NPs are called upon to treat.

Less commonly encountered conditions that are likely to be found on certifying examinations are covered as well. Section V is a basic overview of pacemakers, defibrillators, and cardiac stents. Patient education tips regarding a healthy diet, exercise, tobacco cessation, and stress reduction are provided in a section on *Lifestyles*. The paradigms offered in *Survival Skills* cover such important topics as how to make allies of the nurses and staff, how to handle complicated patients by taking it one step at a time, and the dreaded topic of what to do when you make a mistake. Sample admission orders, discharge summaries, pre- and post-procedure orders and other useful tools for the cardiology PA/NP are provided in the appendix.

Special note to students: *Cardiology Essentials* will make the complex material you learn in the classroom more understandable. It will be invaluable during the family practice and internal medicine rotations, because you will manage many cardiac patients during these rotations. Because cardiology is the most heavily weighted area on the PA-certifying examination, this handbook will help you to prepare. Good luck with your training and preparation for one of the greatest careers imaginable.

Thank you for choosing *Cardiology Essentials*. I hope you find it as enjoyable to read as I found it to write.

Acknowledgments

I am grateful for having had the opportunity to work with and learn from the cardiologists of Wilmington Health Associates and Wilmington Cardiology in Wilmington, North Carolina: Thank you Dr. Helak, Dr. Calhoun, Dr. Everhart, Dr. Brezinski, Dr. Harper, Dr. Richards, Dr. Henry Patel, Dr. Praful Patel, Dr. Murphy, Dr. Lewis, Dr. Weaver, and Dr. Tamisiea. I have also had the pleasure of working with Mary Jackson, ANP; Rebecca Westendorrf, PA-C; and Natalie Jackson, FNP; three extraordinary cardiology providers.

A special thank you to Dr. Savage of Consultants in Cardiology in Roanoke, Virginia for picking up the torch and continuing to keep me up to date with the newest advances in the ever-changing field of cardiology. I am especially grateful for your generosity, which has given me the freedom to pursue my passion for writing.

To the Jefferson College of Health Sciences Physician Assistant Class of 2006 and 2007 (and a little bit of 2008) who inspired me to write this book. I wish you all much success in your professional and personal lives.

Thank you Dave Cella and the staff at Jones and Bartlett for making this book a reality and to Alan Schreiber for all your assistance.

Diagnostic Tools

This section will explain how to perform a cardiac-specific history and physical with attention to the specific historical questions and physical examination findings that are vital in properly evaluating such patients. Tricks for simplifying the interpretation of the 12-lead EKG will be revealed. Finally, an overview of the more commonly utilized cardiac diagnostic studies will be provided with specific information for physician assistants (PAs) and nurse practitioners (NPs) on how to perform several of these studies.

The timely diagnosis of cardiac conditions is crucial if poor outcomes are to be avoided. For example, early identification and management of a myocardial infarction (MI) can help preserve the ejection fraction, which is an important prognostic indicator post-MI. Diagnostic strategies that aid in the timely and accurate diagnosis of cardiac disease are numerous and involve both invasive and noninvasive studies as well as a properly conducted history and physical (H&P) exam.

Chapter 1

Cardiac History and Physical Exam

Introduction

The history and physical exam (simply H&P for short) is a vital part of the cardiac assessment, because it will assist in developing and narrowing down the differential diagnosis. Also, the H&P is a legal document that can be detrimental, if improperly constructed, in the event of a lawsuit. For these reasons, it is important to take the time to learn how to correctly perform and document a cardiac H&P.

First Things First

A legally protective H&P will show the reader that care was taken to inquire about symptoms that might indicate more serious conditions rather than focusing immediately on the most likely diagnosis. This is accomplished by including both pertinent positives and negatives in the history of present illness (HPI) and by conducting a thorough review of systems (ROS).

All positive findings in the H&P must be addressed in the assessment and plan (A/P) so that they do not appear to have been overlooked. If the findings are not a priority, simply state in the A/P that these findings are chronic and stable, are being followed by another medical provider, or will be addressed later.

Prior to performing a complete H&P, it is important to rapidly assess the patient to determine whether the patient is in acute distress or suffering from a life-threatening condition requiring immediate action. A comprehensive H&P can be performed once the patient is stable.

The Cardiac History

Ensure that the patient's name and identifying information are listed on each page with a record of the date and time of the interaction.

History of Present Illness

In the HPI, begin by summarizing the patient's cardiac history, the name of the patient's cardiologist to assure assignment to the correct physician, and how the patient was received.

This introduction assists the person who is reading the note to get an instant feel for the patient so that they can immediately process the forthcoming information and begin to formulate a plan.

Next, summarize the details of the presenting complaint by inquiring about all of the attributes of a symptom. These include:

- location and radiation
- quality
- quantity or severity
- timing including onset, duration, and whether it is continuous or intermittent
- precipitating, exacerbating, or relieving factors
- associated symptoms

Important associated symptoms for cardiac concerns include shortness of breath (SOB), dyspnea on exertion (DOE), orthopnea, paroxysmal nocturnal dyspnea (PND), diaphoresis, nausea, vomiting, palpitations, dizziness, and syncope. Additional symptoms to inquire about will depend on the specific symptom being addressed.

Clarify whether the described symptoms were similar to prior episodes of coronary disease by asking, "Was the pain similar to the pain you experienced prior to your bypass surgery/intervention?" Discover whether nitroglycerine or other medications have been effective and how often they have been required. Assess the level of exertion or the type of activities that have provoked or exacerbated symptoms.

For Example

A 42-year-old male with no prior cardiac history presents to the emergency room (ER) with complaint of chest pain (CP) for 3 days.

or

A 42-year-old male pt of Dr. Heart's with history of coronary heart disease (CHD) s/p coronary artery bypass grafting (CABG) with subsequent drug-eluting stent to the saphenous vein graft (SVG) to the left anterior descending artery (LAD) on 6/26/06 is seen in consultation at the request of Dr. SoSo for evaluation of CP for 3 days.

For Example

A 42-year-old male pt of Dr. Heart's with history of CHD s/p CABG × 4 vessels in 2002 with subsequent drug-eluting stent to the SVG to the LAD on 6/26/06 is seen in consultation at the request of Dr. SoSo for evaluation of CP for 3 days.

Pain is described as anterior precordial tightness/squeezing "like someone is sitting on my chest" and radiates to the neck and left arm. It is a 9/10 in intensity and began 3 days ago while walking the dog. It resolved in 15 minutes with rest, but has recurred with minimal exertion over the past 3 days until this morning when it became continuous since 7 AM when he attempted to walk the dog again. Pain has worsened over the past 4 hours despite the use of nitroglycerine (NTG) sublingual (SL) × 3 and aspirin (ASA) 325 mg orally (po). CP is associated with SOB, diaphoresis, nausea, and palpitations. Denies dizziness, syncope, orthopnea, or PND, but does recall exertional dyspnea over the past 3 or 4 weeks.

Include cardiac risk factors in the last sentence of the HPI when pertinent (such as in a patient with chest pain).

If risk factor information is not pertinent to the chief complaint, it can be placed elsewhere in the H&P. For example, when admitting a patient with an exacerbation of end-stage heart failure, it is better to put the details of her congestive heart failure history and a description of her present symptoms in the HPI and place the risk factors elsewhere in the H&P. In this case, risk factor information is not going to affect the diagnostic strategy or management plan.

Include the patient's response to any treatment performed prior to the performance of the H&P.

For Example

He has a history of hypertension (HTN), but no diabetes mellitus (DM), dyslipidemia, or tobacco abuse. He has no family history (FHx) of early onset CHD, sudden cardiac death, or family members dying young of unknown causes.

For Example

The patient was given ASA 325 mg, and NTG SL × 3 with reduction of his pain from a 9/10 to a 4/10. One inch of nitropaste was then applied and metoprolol 5 mg was administered intravenously (IV) with complete resolution of pain.

Past Medical History

When documenting the past medical history (PMH) in a cardiac patient, it is beneficial to include pertinent negatives in addition to a list of previous illnesses. Include all medical illnesses that are cardiac risk factors if you did not place this information in the HPI.

Additionally, mention whether the patient has had rheumatic fever, because this is an important risk factor for valvular heart disease. Patients who have a history of cancer may have received cardiotoxic chemotherapeutic agents or undergone radiation therapy, which may cause cardiomyopathy. Whether the patient has chronic renal disease is also pertinent in the management and prognosis of cardiac patients and should be questioned. For example, the use of IV contrast during catheterization may worsen renal function.

> **For Example**
> Denies history of hypertension and diabetes; cholesterol status is unknown.

Medications

In addition to the standard list of medications, dosages, and routes of administration, specifically inquire about whether the patient with a history of Coronary Heart Disease has required any nitroglycerine sublingual recently. If the answer is yes, find out how frequently and whether this represents an escalating pattern of usage.

The phosphodiesterase inhibitors sildenafil (Viagra), tadalafil (Cialis), and vardenafil (Levitra) are contraindicated concomitantly with nitrates. It is very important to be aware of their usage in cardiac patients to avoid profound hypotension and therefore worsening ischemia if nitrates are initiated.

Additionally, patients frequently fail to mention over-the-counter (OTC) medications, herbal remedies, and alternative therapies unless specifically asked about them. Pseudoephedrine is a commonly used OTC agent that can worsen hypertension and cause palpitations.

Allergies

In addition to compiling the standard list of drug allergies, ask specifically whether the patient has an allergy to iodine or shellfish, which contains iodine. Iodine is found in the IV contrast that is used during cardiac catheterization.

Document the reaction that resulted from the substance, because many reactions are actually insensitivities or adverse drug reactions rather than true allergies. This distinction may be clinically important. For example, patients who claim to have an aspirin allergy, but simply have had gastrointestinal upset, are usually able to tolerate aspirin after undergoing stent implantation.

Family History

Inquire about cardiac disorders that have a genetic component. These include ischemic heart disease, hypertrophic obstructive cardiomyopathy, Marfan's syndrome (which is often complicated by aortic dissection and mitral valve disease), hemochromatosis (which can lead to cardiomyopathy), and Long QT syndrome (which may result in sudden death). Additionally, familial hypercholesterolemia, hypertension, diabetes mellitus, or homocysteinuria places the patient at risk of premature ischemic heart disease.

Social History

Inquire about the use of cardiotoxic substances such as tobacco, alcohol, illicit drugs, or weight loss agents.

It is important to know what a patient does socially or occupationally because these activities may be affected by the patient's cardiac condition and vice versa. Also, determine who is available as a support system for the patient.

Review of Systems

Listing at least one symptom from each of 10 systems will satisfy billing and coding requirements. If there are no complaints in all systems you can use the phrase, "All systems were reviewed and were negative." However, documenting any pertinent symptoms, both positive and negative, is still essential for proper patient care and protection from litigation.

Pearl

Cocaine use may cause coronary spasm, tachycardia, and increased myocardial oxygen demand leading to ischemia or infarct. Long-term cocaine use may cause dilated cardiomyopathy. The unopposed alpha-adrenergic activity that may occur with the use of beta-blockers is detrimental in these patients, and their use should be avoided.

Other Health Care Providers

Determine the name and contact information of the patient's primary care provider, cardiologist, and cardiac surgeon or electrophysiologist if pertinent.

The Cardiac Physical Exam

Although this section focuses entirely on the cardiovascular system, the physical examination of a cardiac patient involves evaluation of more than just the cardiovascular system. Review the general physical examination elsewhere if needed.

For Example

Constitutional: Denies fatigue (although fatigue is a common complaint that may signify a myriad of conditions, it may be a sign of poor cardiac output, a result of overdiuresis, or a side effect of beta-blocker use), recent weight change (important if you are concerned about acute, decompensated heart failure; unexplained weight loss may indicate an occult malignancy), or fever (helps to distinguish between pneumonia and heart failure).

Skin: Denies diaphoresis (often present in anginal episodes).

Head, Eyes, Ears, Nose, Throat (HEENT): Denies recent vision changes (important to assess in patients on amiodarone therapy).

Neurological: Denies headache (which may be associated with hypertensive crisis and is also a common adverse effect of nitrates and calcium channel blockers).

Respiratory: Denies dyspnea or cough (or write "see HPI" if you already addressed this).

Cardiac: See HPI.

Gastrointestinal: Denies hematochezia or melena (melena, the presence of black, tarry-looking stool, indicates the possibility of an upper GI bleed and should be a part of your ROS if you are considering the use of antiplatelets or anticoagulants).

Urinary: Denies hematuria (important to assess for any bleeding problems if anticoagulants are to be instituted) or change in urinary frequency; denies history of renal disease.

Genitourinary: Denies sexual dysfunction (which is a common vascular problem that may coexist with other vascular disorders and is a possible adverse effect of beta-blocker therapy).

Endocrine: Denies temperature intolerance (thyroid abnormalities can be an adverse effect of amiodarone [Cordarone/ Pacerone] therapy or may be the underlying reason for cardiac disease); denies polyphagia, polyuria, or polydipsia (may indicate diabetes mellitus).

Hematologic: Denies easy bleeding or bruising (may indicate a coagulation disorder).

Vascular: Denies history of a transient ischemic attack (TIA) or stroke. Denies one-sided weakness, slurred speech, or visual disturbances. Denies history of peripheral vascular disease or symptoms of intermittent claudication (other vascular disorders often coexist with CHD).

Vital Signs

Although the vital signs are frequently performed by other personnel, be prepared to repeat blood pressure (BP) readings when they appear abnormal or if you are concerned about incorrect technique. Although the heart rate and rhythm are frequently documented in the chart, the amplitude and contour of the arterial pulse will need to be assessed later when the carotid arteries are examined.

Jugular Venous Pressure (JVP)

Elevate the head of the bed to 30 degrees and locate the highest point of pulsation of the internal jugular vein. Measure the vertical distance from this point to the sternal angle. The JVP is considered elevated if this distance is greater than 3–4 centimeters.

Carotid Arteries

Prior to auscultating the carotid arteries for bruits, palpate the amplitude and contour of the arterial pulse. A normal carotid pulse will have a rapid, smooth upstroke followed by a more gradual downstroke with an amplitude that is neither weak nor bounding. This may sound difficult to assess, but if you palpate numerous normal carotid arteries, an abnormality will become immediately apparent.

Inspection and Palpation

Perform a general inspection of the patient for signs of distress such as cyanosis, retraction, excessive use of accessory muscles of respiration, or tachypnea.

Inspect the chest wall for abnormalities such as pectus excavatum, which is a depression in the lower portion of the sternum that may compress cardiac structures leading to murmurs.

Locate the point of maximal impulse (PMI), the apex of the heart, by placing the palm of your hand by the axilla and moving anteriorly until the PMI is localized. If it is larger than a quarter in diameter, note that it is diffuse. Describe its location by noting its position relative to the midclavicular, midsternal, or midaxillary line.

> **For Example**
>
> The PMI is palpated 2 cm lateral to the midclavicular line

The right ventricle sits anteriorly in the chest cavity with the left ventricle situated behind it and at the apex. Palpate for a right ventricular heave by placing the palm of your hand firmly upon the left lower sternal border. A right ventricular heave may indicate pulmonary stenosis or pulmonary hypertension. A *heave* is a rising of the chest wall that is palpable.

Palpate for thrills over the aortic (second right intercostal space) and pulmonic (second left intercostal space) areas. An aortic thrill is a sign of aortic stenosis and a pulmonic thrill is a sign of pulmonary hypertension. A *thrill* is a humming vibration like the way a cat's throat feels while it is purring.

Palpate over the chest wall and over the costochondral areas to assess for tenderness.

Auscultation

Normal Heart Sounds (S1 and S2)

The mitral valve, which sits between the left atrium and left ventricle, closes when preparing to eject blood out of the left ventricle to prevent blood from backing up into the atrium. S1 is the sound you hear when the mitral valve closes and it marks the beginning of systole.

S2, the sound you hear when the aortic valve closes, marks the beginning of diastole. When the aortic valve closes, the mitral valve opens and the left ventricle is allowed to fill with blood.

Splitting of the Heart Sounds

While the first heart sound (S1) and the second heart sound (S2) represent the sounds of the left-sided valves, what is going on in the right side of the heart? The right side of the heart involves much less pressure, because it only has to push the blood to the lungs instead of all the way around the body, so the heart sounds are not as loud and may be inaudible. The right-sided valves close slightly after the left-sided valves. For this reason, you may hear two sounds for the S1 and the S2, but they are so close together that it sounds like a splitting of the sound rather than a completely distinct sound.

Therefore, while listening to the S1, you may actually hear the mitral valve closing first and then the much softer tricuspid valve closing. This is very difficult to hear and it is more common to hear the S2 splitting rather than the S1.

The S2 represents the closure of the aortic valve (A2) as well as the closure of the pulmonic valve (P2), which is softer and is slightly delayed. Normally the splitting of the S2 is only audible during inspiration. This is thought to be because the increased lung volumes during inspiration prolong the ejection of blood from the right ventricle and thereby delay the closure of the pulmonic valve. This is a normal physiological occurrence. Auscultate over the pulmonic area during inspiration to hear a split S2.

Pathological Splitting of the Heart Sounds

Paradoxical splitting means that the aortic valve closes after the pulmonic valve rather than the other way around. This delay in closure of the aortic valve is most commonly due to a left bundle branch block. If paradoxical splitting of the S2 were to occur, you would hear the soft component of the S2 prior to the loud component.

Wide splitting of the S2 may occur in any condition that further delays the closure of the pulmonic valve (i.e., pulmonic stenosis or right bundle branch block) or any condition that causes early closure of the aortic valve (i.e., mitral regurgitation).

Fixed splitting occurs when the split occurs during both inspiration and expiration. Splitting of the heart sounds during expiration is abnormal and may signify right ventricular failure or an atrial septal defect.

Abnormal Heart Sounds

A systolic click is high pitched and usually occurs in mid-to-late systole. It usually signifies mitral valve prolapse.

An opening snap (OS) is an abnormal sound that occurs when the motion of the mitral valve is restricted as it is opening. This may occur in mitral stenosis.

An S3, sometimes called a *gallop*, may be physiologic in children and young adults. In older adults, it is highly suggestive of ventricular volume overload due to CHF or valvular heart disease such as mitral regurgitation. The S3 is audible during rapid ventricular filling, which occurs immediately following the S2.

An S4 (or atrial gallop) represents atrial contraction; therefore, you will hear an S4 just prior to the S1. This is when the atrium contracts to fill the ventricle with its remaining blood just before the mitral valve closes and systole begins. An S4 may be heard in healthy adults but is commonly heard in patients with hypertension.

Both extra heart sounds, the S3 and S4, are dull, low-pitched sounds that are best heard with the bell placed at the apex with the patient in the left lateral decubitus position.

> **Bottom Line**
>
> Both the S3 and S4 are audible after the S2 and before the subsequent S1. The S3, however, occurs immediately after the S2, whereas the S4 occurs much closer to the subsequent S1.

Heart Murmurs

A murmur has a longer duration than the heart sounds just described. It is caused by turbulent blood flow and may be physiologic, as in young people or pregnancy, or pathologic, as in valvular heart disease.

A stenotic valve means that the lumen or opening of the valve has become narrowed and the flow of blood through the valve is impeded. A regurgitant or incompetent valve is one that cannot close completely, thereby allowing blood to leak backwards (retrograde blood flow).

Murmurs are described by their quality, intensity, location, radiation, timing, and what maneuvers make them more audible.

Quality

Not all murmurs sound the same. Some murmurs peak earlier in the cardiac cycle than others; some murmurs are continuous and don't peak at all. These differences are described as the quality of the murmur and help to illicit the etiology of the murmur.

A crescendo-decrescendo murmur peaks near midsystole and usually stops before the S2. This gap between the murmur and the S2 is the best way to differentiate these murmurs from holosystolic murmurs, which are present throughout systole. Crescendo-decrescendo murmurs are typical of aortic stenosis and hypertrophic obstructive cardiomyopathy (HOCM).

Holosystolic murmurs begin immediately at S1 and continue right up to the S2. They are pathologic and occur when blood passes from a high-pressure chamber to a low-pressure chamber through a valve or other structure that should be closed. This may occur in mitral regurgitation, tricuspid regurgitation, or a ventricular septal defect.

Intensity

Murmurs are graded on a scale from 1 to 6. A grade 1 murmur requires concentration to hear. A grade 2 murmur is heard immediately upon positioning your stethoscope in the correct location, but is quiet. A grade 3 murmur is moderately loud.

Pearl

A thrill may be palpated at the area where a murmur is heard. If you feel a thrill, then the murmur is classified as a grade 4/6 or greater.

By definition, if you claim that a murmur is louder than a grade 3, you must palpate a thrill in addition to hearing the murmur. A grade 4 murmur is loud with a palpable thrill. A grade 5 murmur is loud enough to hear with the stethoscope partially off the chest and has a palpable thrill. A grade 6 murmur has a palpable thrill and may be heard with the stethoscope entirely off the chest.

Location

As you inch the stethoscope over the chest, be aware of what structures you are auscultating. The usual auscultation sequence is as follows: First, listen to the aortic region at the second right intercostal space (ICS), followed by the pulmonic region at the second left ICS, next the tricuspid region at the left lower sternal border, and finally the mitral region, which is located at the apex.

Radiation

Whether a murmur radiates may help decipher its etiology or determine the severity of a valvular disorder. *Aortic sclerosis,* the stiffening of the aortic valve due to advanced age, has a similar sounding murmur to aortic stenosis, but does not radiate to the carotids or obscure the sound of the S2. Aortic stenosis (AS), when it becomes more severe, may obliterate the S2 and radiate to the carotid arteries.

Timing

Focus on active auscultation. In other words, try not to daydream while listening! If you hear a murmur, determine whether it is present during systole or diastole. Systolic murmurs occur when the blood is being pumped out of the heart so the aortic valve must be open and the mitral valve must be closed. What kind of valve disorder can you have when the aortic valve is open? It must be some kind of obstruction that is impeding the flow of blood through the open aortic valve such as aortic stenosis. What kind of valve disorder can you have if the mitral valve is closed? It must be a leaky valve or regurgitation through the closed mitral valve as in mitral regurgitation (MR). The same principles apply to the right-sided structures.

In diastole, the heart relaxes and the blood exits the atria to fill the ventricles. This means that the aortic valve is closed and the mitral valve is open. A diastolic murmur, therefore, must indicate a regurgitant aortic valve or an obstructed or stenotic mitral valve. Again, these principles also apply to the right-sided structures.

> **Bottom Line**
> Systolic murmurs include aortic stenosis and mitral regurgitation.

> **Bottom Line**
> Diastolic murmurs may include aortic insufficiency (regurgitation) or mitral stenosis.

Maneuvers

Squatting increases venous return to the heart, which increases the volume of blood in the ventricle. This increase in blood volume worsens the murmur of AS by increasing the amount of blood that cannot pass through a stenotic valve.

Squatting reduces the murmur of HOCM because the increased blood volume pushes the hypertrophied ventricular wall out of the way of the outflow tract, thereby decreasing the amount of obstruction. The increased blood volume caused by squatting also reduces the murmur of mitral valve prolapse (MVP) by reducing the amount of prolapse.

> **Bottom Line**
>
> Squatting worsens the murmur of AS and improves the murmur of HOCM and MVP. The Valsalva maneuver worsens the murmur of HOCM and MVP and improves the murmur of AS. This is because one of these maneuvers (squatting) increases the volume of blood in the ventricle and the other maneuver (Valsalva) decreases the ventricular volume.

The Valsalva maneuver decreases venous return to the heart (preload), thereby reducing the left ventricular volume. If there is less blood to pump out of the heart, then the murmur will not be as loud as the blood passes through a stenotic aortic valve. Hence, the Valsalva maneuver decreases the murmur of AS.

On the other hand, if you have a hypertrophied ventricle that is obstructing the outflow tract, less blood volume in the ventricle means that the hypertrophied ventricular wall will overly the outflow tract even more. Therefore, the Valsalva maneuver will worsen the murmur of HOCM.

To perform the Valsalva maneuver, simply ask the patient to bear down as if they are trying to have a bowel movement. Alternatively, place your hand on the patient's abdomen while they are supine and ask them to strain against it.

Heart Rub

A pericardial friction rub, which occurs in pericarditis, is a continuous murmur. This means that it is audible in both systole and diastole. It is a high-pitched scraping or scratching sound that is best heard with the diaphragm. It may be more audible during exhalation and with the patient leaning forward.

TABLE 1.1   Auscultation of Common Heart Murmurs and Extra Sounds

Murmur or Heart Sound	Listen with	During	Tips
Aortic stenosis	Diaphragm	Expiration	May radiate to carotids
Aortic regurgitation	Diaphragm	Expiration	Have patient lean forward
Mitral stenosis	Bell	Expiration	Place patient in left lateral position
Mitral regurgitation	Diaphragm	n/a	May radiate to axilla
S3	Bell	n/a	Place patient in left lateral position
S4	Bell	n/a	Place patient in left lateral position

Pearl

An acronym for remembering how to best auscultate for mitral stenosis is "**BELL**": Listen with the **B**ell during **E**xpiration in the **L**eft **L**ateral decubitus position.

For Example

Documenting a cardiovascular exam:

General: Describe the patient's general appearance. Some adjectives you may choose include the following: well-appearing, cachectic, frail, appears older than stated age, no apparent distress (NAD), pleasant, anxious, alert, obtunded, sedated, awakens only to painful stimuli (i.e., rubbing over the sternum), seated in chair reading a book.

VS: Document the blood pressure, pulse, respiration, and weight; include orthostatic BP, BP in both arms, temperature, body mass index or waist circumference, and/or pulse oximetry when appropriate.

Skin: Descriptors include warm and dry, diaphoretic, cyanotic, acrocyanosis, pale, or gray (a gray complexion is particularly ominous).

Eyes: Document arcus senilis (a thin grayish white arc or circle around the perimeter of the cornea; which may signify hyperlipidemia in younger people and is a common normal finding in the elderly), xanthelasma (slightly raised yellowish plaques found around the nasal portions of the eyelids; may indicate hyperlipidemia), and pale conjunctiva if indicated.

Neck: Document JVP, the nature of the carotid upstrokes, and whether carotid bruits were audible.

Lungs: Describe breath sounds as normal or diminished and note whether any adventitious sounds (i.e., wheezes, rhonchi, or rales) were audible.

Cardiac: Document the location of the PMI and whether heaves or thrills were present. Describe the quality of the S1 and S2 (i.e., normal S1 and S2 or prosthetic-sounding heart sounds). Describe any murmurs, gallops, or rubs if present.

Abdomen: Document ascites, hepatomegaly, hepatojugular reflux (HJR), or bruits if noted on exam.

Vascular: Document the quality of the femoral and distal pulses and note whether they are bilaterally equal. Document pedal edema, venous stasis changes, or arterial insufficiency changes.

BACK TO THE BASICS

Bisferiens pulse: the arterial pulse has two systolic peaks. This may indicate aortic regurgitation.

Dextrocardia: the heart is located on the right side of the body. This is usually associated with congenital heart disease.

Janeway lesions: nontender, hemorrhagic lesions on the palms and soles. May be present in endocarditis.

Left lateral decubitus position: have the patient lie on their left side with their left arm under their head and their right arm at their side. They can bend their right knee for comfort. Use this position to hear mitral murmurs better. As you gently press the patient's right shoulder forward, you can auscultate the mitral region while the apex of the heart falls closer to the chest wall.

Orthostatic hypotension: a drop in systolic blood pressure of greater than 20 mmHg when the patient goes from a recumbent to a standing position.

Osler's nodes: tender, purple nodules on the fingerpads. May be present in endocarditis.

Pulsus paradoxis: a decrease in the blood pressure on inspiration compared to expiration (by >10mmHg). This may be caused by cardiac tamponade, constrictive pericarditis, or obstructive airway disease.

Pulsus alternans: Palpate the radial (or femoral) artery for alternating strong and weak pulses. This may signify left heart failure.

Situs inversus: the heart, liver, and stomach are all located on the opposite side of the body.

Splinter hemorrhages: red or brown linear streaks in the nail bed. May be present in endocarditis, but also occur without any known cause.

Thrill: a humming vibration on the chest wall, like the purring of a cat, which is palpable.

Valsalva Maneuver: Ask the patient to bear down as if straining to have a bowel movement or place your hand on their abdomen and ask them to strain against your hand. This decreases blood return to the right side of the heart and results in a subsequent fall in left ventricular volume and, therefore, blood pressure.

Waterhammer pulse: a strong, high volume pulse that quickly collapses. It is classically associated with aortic regurgitation (AR).

Chapter 2

EKG Tricks

Introduction

After completing the history and physical exam, an electrocardiogram (EKG) is often obtained. By measuring the electrical activity in the heart, the EKG may be the first indicator of ischemia, electrolyte abnormalities, adverse drug effects, or structural changes in the heart.

BACK TO THE BASICS

Basic EKG Components
The basic components of the EKG are labeled in **Figure 2.1**. The p wave represents atrial depolarization. The PR interval represents depolarization delay in the atrioventricular (AV) node and is measured from the beginning of the p wave to the beginning of the QRS complex. The QRS complex denotes ventricular depolarization. A downward deflection during ventricular depolarization is described as a Q wave, whereas an upward deflection is referred to as an R wave. A negative deflection that has been preceded by another downward deflection is called an S wave. It is perfectly normal to see all or some of these components on the EKG depending on which lead you are looking at. The point where the QRS complex terminates is called the j point. The ST segment, which begins at the j point and ends at the beginning of the t wave, signifies the state of electrical neutrality that exists between ventricular depolarization and repolarization. Ventricular repolarization is represented by the t wave. The electrical denotation of ventricular systole runs from the beginning of the QRS complex through the end of the t wave and is called the QT interval.

(continues)

BACK TO THE BASICS (continued)

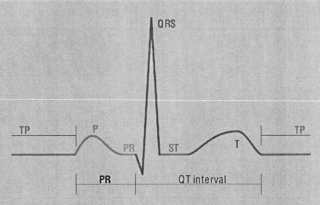

FIGURE 2.1 Basic Components of the EKG

Source: Garcia, Tomas B., and Neil E. Holtz. *12-Lead ECG: The Art of Interpretation.* Jones and Bartlett Publishers. 2001.

Normal Pacemaker Activity and Automaticity

The sinoatrial (SA) node is the normal pacemaker of the heart; if it cannot function, then other areas of the heart will step in to fire automatically, hence the term automaticity. Automaticity is the heart's own intrinsic back-up system because if the heart doesn't beat, death is a certainty. Sometimes these other areas decide to fire despite a normally functioning SA node, resulting in premature beats or arrhythmias.

The AV node allows for a slight delay to allow time for all the signals from the atrium to arrive, so that the impulse can be propagated through the His-Purkinje system all at once. This enables the ventricular cells to depolarize more efficiently and cohesively resulting in a narrow QRS. Excluding conduction delays such as bundle branch blocks, preexcitation syndromes, and paced rhythms, a widened QRS is initiated by an impulse that originated below (or after) the AV node. Otherwise the impulse would have passed through the AV node, waited for all the signals from the atrium to arrive, and then efficiently conducted a nice, narrow QRS complex by sending the impulse through the His-Purkinje system all at once.

Atrial cells can conduct at a faster heart rate than the other cardiac cells and are usually first to initiate an impulse when the SA node fails. If atrial cells other than the SA node initiate the impulse, then p waves will be present but they may have a different axis or morphology because the electrical signal is traveling from elsewhere within the atrium.

(continues)

If the atrial cells don't initiate a heart beat, the junction is the next candidate. The junction is where the AV node is located. These cells propagate at a slower rate than the atrial cells, but still utilize the His-Purkinje system, allowing for an efficient ventricular depolarization. Hence, a nice narrow QRS is

generated, but at a slower ventricular rate than an impulse generated from atrial cells. If the junction doesn't initiate an impulse, the ventricular cells may. Unfortunately, the ventricular cells fire at a very slow rate and are very inefficient at conducting the impulse throughout the ventricles. This is because they have to propagate from cell to cell rather than by utilizing the super-efficient His-Purkinje system. For this reason, ventricular escape rhythms, which rely on the automaticity of ventricular cells to sustain a heart rhythm, are slow and have a wide complex QRS (**Figure 2.2**).

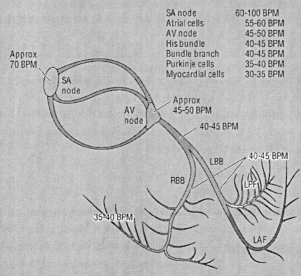

SA node	60-100 BPM
Atrial cells	55-60 BPM
AV node	45-50 BPM
His bundle	40-45 BPM
Bundle branch	40-45 BPM
Purkinje cells	35-40 BPM
Myocardial cells	30-35 BPM

FIGURE 2.2 Myocardial Conduction System

Source: Garcia, Tomas B., and Neil E. Holtz. *12-Lead ECG: The Art of Interpretation.* Jones and Bartlett Publishers. 2001.

First Things First

Before interpreting an EKG, confirm the patient's name and date, ensure the speed and magnitude are on the correct setting, and try to locate an old EKG for comparison. The speed should be set at 25 mm/sec and the magnitude or gain should be set at 10 mm/mV. This is represented by a bar at the end of each line on one side of the EKG, which should be two large boxes high.

Cardio Reality

While performing a site visit, a second-year physician assistant student presented a patient with dyspnea on exertion (DOE) to me. He astutely ordered an EKG, which revealed a left bundle branch block (BBB) and correctly determined that he would be unable to evaluate for ST-t wave abnormalities in this patient. Because the student was concerned about the possibility of heart failure, the patient was scheduled for an echocardiogram.

As we discussed the case, I flipped through the patient's chart and noticed that a prior EKG did not reveal a bundle branch block. Once we had this new information, we were more concerned about the possibility of ischemia. You see, if the BBB had been present in a previous EKG it would have been a nonspecific finding. However, because it was a new finding, an ischemic etiology was a strong possibility. The new information gleaned from the old EKG was very helpful in determining the appropriate management strategy for the patient.

To avoid overlooking valuable EKG clues, use a systematic approach when interpreting an EKG. First, determine the rate and rhythm. Next, determine whether there is axis deviation, which should raise the suspicion of other EKG abnormalities such as a bundle branch block or ventricular hypertrophy. Finally, assess each interval and complex.

Rate

There are two ways to look at an EKG and instantly determine the heart rate. The simplest method involves looking down at the paper, locating the QRS complex that is closest to a dark vertical line, then counting either forward or backward to the same point on the adjacent QRS complex. For each large box you pass, select the next number off the mnemonic "300-150-100-75-60-50" to estimate the rate in beats per minute (bpm) (**Figure 2.3**).

This method is not useful in bradycardia or if the rhythm is irregular. In these instances, you simply count the number of complexes in a period of time and multiply by the amount of time necessary to equal 60 seconds. Each small box represents 0.04 seconds and each large box represents 0.2 seconds. Therefore, five large boxes represent a 1-second strip. Most people use a 6-second strip, which is 30 large boxes, because

Pearl

There are approximately 50 large boxes on the rhythm strip of a 12-lead EKG. Remember that 50 large boxes = 10 seconds. All you have to do is count the number of QRS complexes on the EKG rhythm strip and multiply by 6. You don't even need to measure an interval to count!

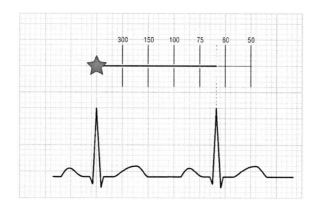

FIGURE 2.3 Easy Method for Assessing Heart Rate

Source: Garcia, Tomas B., and Neil E. Holtz. *12-Lead ECG: The Art of Interpretation.* Jones and Bartlett Publishers. 2001.

it is easy to multiply by 10. Simply count the number of QRS complexes in those 30 large boxes and then multiply the number of complexes by 10. That is your rate in beats per minute.

Rhythm

Determining the rhythm is easier if the following questions are addressed methodically:

1. Is there a p wave before every QRS?
2. Is there a QRS following every p wave?
3. Is the rhythm regular or irregular?
4. Is the QRS narrow or wide?
5. Is the rate too fast or too slow?

Sinus Rhythm

Sinus rhythm implies that the SA node initiated the impulse. Sinus rhythm exists when the following criteria are met: there is a p wave preceding every QRS, a QRS following every p wave, and the p waves have a normal morphology (upright in leads I, II, and III) (**Figure 2.4**).

Once the rhythm is identified as "sinus," distinguish between normal sinus rhythm (NSR), sinus bradycardia, and sinus tachycardia by assessing the rate.

A sinus rhythm with a rate less than 60 bpm is sinus bradycardia, which may be caused by certain medications (i.e., digoxin, beta-blockers, diltiazem, verapamil, or amiodarone). Atropine or cardiac pacing may be necessary in acute episodes of symptomatic bradycardia. If no reversible cause is identified and the patient is symptomatic, a permanent pacemaker may be required.

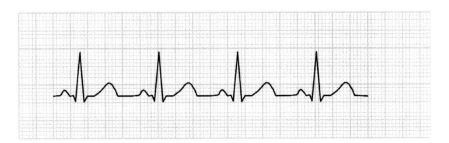

FIGURE 2.4   Normal Sinus Rhythm

Source: Garcia, Tomas B., and Neil E. Holtz. 12-Lead ECG: The Art of Interpretation. Jones and Bartlett Publishers. 2001.

If the rate is greater than 100 bpm, sinus tachycardia is present. Sinus tachycardia is a normal physiologic response to underlying problems such as anemia, dehydration, anxiety, pain, fever, hypovolemia, myocardial infarction, or hypoxia. Management is geared toward treating the underlying condition. Sinus tachycardia secondary to hyperthyroidism is managed with a beta-blocker until the underlying disease is controlled.

Inappropriate sinus tachycardia may be present if the resting heart rate is greater than 100 in the absence of an identifiable cause or structural heart disease. Treatment with a beta-blocker or verapamil may be considered.

Sinus arrhythmia is a sinus rhythm with a rate that fluctuates cyclically with respiration. It is frequently seen in children and may also be found in healthy adults (**Figure 2.5**).

Bottom Line

Rhythms that originate from the SA node (Sinus Rhythms)

Normal sinus rhythm	Regular rhythm, regular rate (60–100 bpm)
Sinus bradycardia	Regular rhythm, slow rate (<60 bpm)
Sinus tachycardia	Regular rhythm, rapid rate (>100 bpm)
Sinus arrhythmia	Irregular rhythm, regular rate

Premature Atrial Contractions

Premature atrial contractions (PACs) are ectopic beats initiated from within the atrium. They may occur individually, in pairs (couplets), or in trios (triplets). They may also occur in a rhythmic sequence alternating with a normal beat. This is called bigeminy if every other beat is prematurely contracted and trigeminy if every third beat is prematurely contracted. PACs present as a narrow complex QRS preceded by a premature p wave. Although therapy is seldom necessary, a beta-blocker may be considered in symptomatic patients.

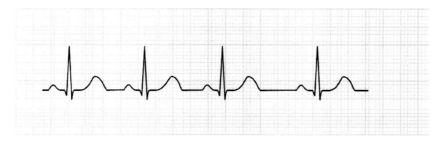

FIGURE 2.5 Sinus Arrhythmia

Source: Garcia, Tomas B., and Neil E. Holtz. 12-Lead ECG: The Art of Interpretation. Jones and Bartlett Publishers. 2001.

Ectopic Atrial Rhythm

An ectopic atrial rhythm is a regular rhythm with a normal rate that arises from an area within the atrium other than the SA node. The rhythm is almost indistinguishable from sinus rhythm aside from abnormal p wave morphology.

Paroxysmal Atrial Tachycardia

In paroxysmal atrial tachycardia (PAT), the rate is rapid and the rhythm is regular; it is the rapid version of an ectopic atrial rhythm. If p waves are present, they may appear abnormal or inverted because these atrial impulses are arising outside of the SA node (**Figure 2.6**).

Wandering Atrial Pacemaker

In a wandering atrial pacemaker (WAP), the rate is normal but the rhythm is irregular. There may be a p wave for every QRS and vice versa, but there are at least three different kinds of p waves noted. These atrial impulses are arising in the atrium from several different locations (**Figure 2.7**).

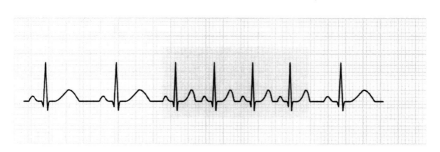

FIGURE 2.6 Paroxysmal Atrial Tachycardia

Source: Garcia, Tomas B., and Neil E. Holtz. 12-Lead ECG: The Art of Interpretation. Jones and Bartlett Publishers. 2001.

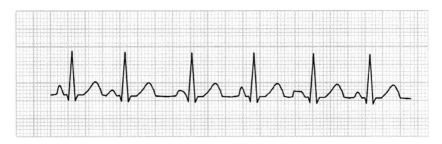

FIGURE 2.7 Wandering Atrial Pacemaker
Source: Garcia, Tomas B., and Neil E. Holtz. 12-Lead ECG: The Art of Interpretation. Jones and Bartlett Publishers. 2001.

Multifocal Atrial Tachycardia

In multifocal atrial tachycardia (MAT), the rate is rapid but the rhythm is irregular. This rhythm is the same as in the WAP, except the rate is rapid. Chronic obstructive pulmonary disease (COPD) is a common cause of MAT. Because it is a fast and irregular rhythm, MAT is often confused with atrial fibrillation. However, if you look carefully, you will clearly detect p waves and they will have at least three different morphologies. Treatment is geared toward management of underlying COPD and hypoxia (**Figure 2.8**).

Atrial Fibrillation

The rhythm is irregularly irregular in atrial fibrillation (AF). The atria are quivering rather than contracting so p waves are not discernible as shown in **Figure 2.9**. The rate may be fast, normal, or slow depending on the number of impulses that conduct through the AV node. Management is discussed in Chapter 21.

Pearl

SVT with aberrancy, sometimes called Ashman's phenomenon, is a wide complex SVT that may be difficult to distinguish from ventricular tachycardia (VT). If you are unsure, treat it as a wide complex tachycardia, which is essentially treating the patient as if they have VT.

Supraventricular Tachycardia

Supraventricular tachycardia (SVT) is a collection of arrhythmias that originate somewhere above the ventricles, hence the name. In SVT, the rhythm is regular and the rate is rapid. Because the depolarization conducts through the normal His-Purkinje system, the QRS will appear narrow unless aberrant conduction exists (such as in patients with concomitant bundle branch blocks).

Initial management of stable patients with SVT includes vagal maneuvers such as carotid sinus massage or Valsalva maneuvers such as asking

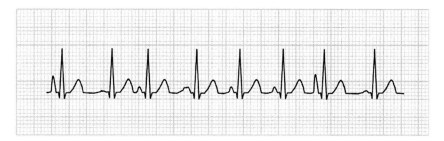

FIGURE 2.8 Multifocal Atrial Tachycardia

Source: Garcia, Tomas B., and Neil E. Holtz. 12-Lead ECG: The Art of Interpretation. Jones and Bartlett Publishers. 2001.

Advanced Concept

AV nodal reentrant tachycardia (AVNRT), the most common type of SVT, involves two pathways of conduction linking the atria to the ventricles rather than one. One of these pathways conducts rapidly while the other conducts slowly. Often a PAC will place one pathway in a refractory period, allowing the secondary pathway to take over. Once this secondary pathway spreads the impulse from the atrium to the ventricle, it may then conduct retrograde over the first pathway, which is no longer in refractory mode. This causes a reentrant circuit.

AV reentrant tachycardia (AVRT) differs from AVNRT by having an accessory pathway that is located outside of the AV node. AVRT has one pathway that conducts from the atria to the ventricles through the AV node and another pathway (the accessory pathway) that conducts around the AV node. Wolff-Parkinson-White syndrome is one example of AVRT. Atrial flutter, another type of SVT, is discussed later.

If patients with SVT are clinically stable, take the time to try to further classify the rhythm. In AVNRT, p waves will be buried within the QRS or retrograde p waves may be seen slurring the terminal portion of the QRS. In AVRT, retrograde p waves may be visible after the QRS.

If impulses are initiated in the atrium, as in atrial flutter and atrial tachycardia, then blocking the AV node will not affect the p waves but will slow the ventricular rate unmasking the underlying p waves. These rhythms will not be terminated by blocking AV conduction because they do not rely on the AV node for perpetuation of the circuit. The circuit is located in the atrium and as soon as the AV node is no longer blocked the arrhythmia will continue.

Both AVNRT and AVRT rely on the AV node for perpetuation of the reentrant circuit and, therefore, blocking AV nodal conduction may successfully terminate these rhythms.

Blocking the AV node can be accomplished by performing vagal maneuvers such as carotid sinus massage or by administering adenosine as a rapid IV push (6 mg followed by 12 mg if necessary).

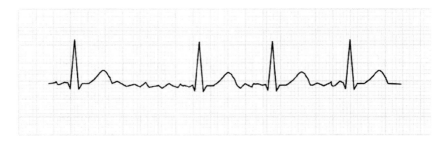

FIGURE 2.9 Atrial Fibrillation
Source: Garcia, Tomas B., and Neil E. Holtz. 12-Lead ECG: The Art of Interpretation. Jones and Bartlett Publishers. 2001.

the patient to bear down as if having a bowel movement. If such maneuvers fail, rapid IV push of adenosine can be given acutely. Chronic therapy involves radiofrequency ablation or medical management with AV nodal blocking agents such as beta-blockers, diltiazem, verapamil, or digoxin.

If patients are hypotensive, have acute mental status changes, or are suffering from chest pain or dyspnea, they may be unstable and should be treated with immediate cardioversion per advance cardiac life support (ACLS) protocol.

Atrial Flutter

In atrial flutter, the atria are contracting regularly at about 300 beats per minute and the p waves have a sawtooth appearance. The AV node cannot conduct this rapidly so only some impulses pass through to the ventricle. Ventricular rate is determined by the degree of AV block, which may be variable. If the AV block is variable, the ventricular rhythm may be irregular. A 2:1 block may be mistaken for sinus tachycardia because the rhythm appears regular at approximately 150 bpm (**Figure 2.10**).

Atrial flutter is managed much the same as atrial fibrillation. Catheter ablation is an effective means of definitive management.

Pearl

Be cautious of a heart rate of about 150 beats per minute. Although a heart rate of approximately 150 beats per minute may be sinus tachycardia, always consider the possibility of atrial flutter. Look at the p waves in leads V1 and II very carefully. Consider carotid sinus massage to slow the rate of conduction and see if flutter waves appear on the tracing. Always listen for carotid bruits prior to performing carotid sinus massage; you don't want to dislodge a clot and cause a stroke.

Junctional Rhythm

A junctional rhythm is regular with a rate between 40–60 bpm. The impulse arises from the AV node; therefore, there are no p waves discernible unless they are retrograde. Retrograde p waves will be inverted and may be seen before or after the QRS complex. Because the impulse still conducts through the His-Purkinje system, the QRS appears narrow and normal (**Figure 2.11**).

A pacemaker may be necessary if the patient becomes symptomatic from decreased cardiac output.

Ventricular Rhythms

Ventricular rhythms arise from the ventricle; therefore, there are no p waves. The QRS appears widened because the impulses are not efficiently conducted through the His-Purkinje system. These rhythms have different names based on how fast or slow they are. An idioventricular rhythm is a regular rhythm at about 30–40 bpm, whereas an accelerated idioventricular rhythm (AIVR) is a similar rhythm with a rate that is faster than the idioventricular rate but slower than ventricular tachycardia, which is typically 100–120 bpm or faster.

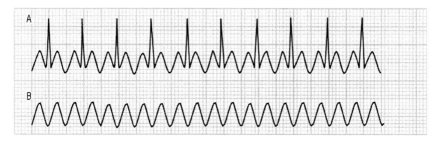

FIGURE 2.10 Atrial Flutter with 2:1 Block

Source: Garcia, Tomas B., and Neil E. Holtz. 12-Lead ECG: The Art of Interpretation. Jones and Bartlett Publishers. 2001.

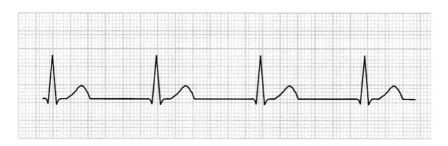

FIGURE 2.11 Junctional Rhythm

Source: Garcia, Tomas B., and Neil E. Holtz. 12-Lead ECG: The Art of Interpretation. Jones and Bartlett Publishers. 2001.

AIVRs are seen almost exclusively in the setting of reperfusion of ischemic myocardium, but may also accompany electrolyte abnormalities such as hypokalemia, digoxin toxicity, or hypoxia. Treatment is rarely necessary, but if patients are unstable or symptomatic atropine or atrial pacing can be considered. These modalities will stimulate the sinus rhythm to speed up and override the ectopic ventricular focus.

Bottom Line

Ventricular Rhythms

Idioventricular rhythm	Slow (30–40 bpm)
Accelerated idioventricular rhythm	Normal (40–100 bpm)
Ventricular tachycardia	Rapid (greater than 100–120 bpm)

Cardio Reality

I remember the first time I saw a wide-complex tachycardia. The patient's nurse called me to the telemetry floor. She showed me the telemetry strip, which revealed a long row of wide QRS complexes. I became nervous because I thought I was looking at ventricular tachycardia. The nurse calmly stated, "It looks like an idioventricular rhythm." This well-respected cardiac nurse's confidence in her interpretation calmed me down long enough to realize that the ventricular rate was only about 40 bpm. I had never even heard the term idioventricular rhythm before, but now I will never forget it. Thank goodness for nurses and thank goodness I held my tongue long enough to benefit from her expertise and discover what was going on!

Premature Ventricular Contractions

Premature ventricular contractions (PVCs) are ectopic ventricular beats that are wide complex and are not preceded by a p wave. First determine the underlying rhythm and then identify any premature (ectopic) beats that may be present. For example, you may have normal sinus rhythm with PVCs. If all of the ectopic beats look the same, they are called unifocal; if there are different morphologies of ectopic beats they are called multifocal. This indicates that they are originating from more than one focus within the ventricle (**Figure 2.12**).

PVCs are often benign and may be aggravated by stress, caffeine, nicotine, alcohol, or sympathomimetics such as are often found in OTC cold medications. If PVCs are infrequent, asymptomatic, and occur in the setting of normal cardiac function, then no treatment is required, If PVCs are frequent, ensure that potassium and magnesium levels are not low. Beta-blockers may be considered for symptomatic relief.

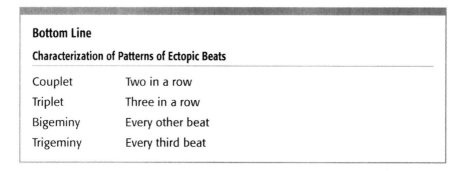

Bottom Line

Characterization of Patterns of Ectopic Beats

Couplet	Two in a row
Triplet	Three in a row
Bigeminy	Every other beat
Trigeminy	Every third beat

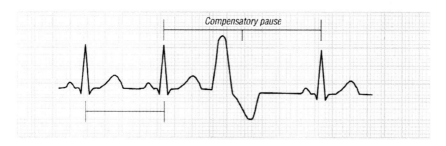

FIGURE 2.12   Premature Ventricular Contractions

Source: Garcia, Tomas B., and Neil E. Holtz. 12-Lead ECG: The Art of Interpretation. Jones and Bartlett Publishers. 2001.

Ventricular Tachycardia

In ventricular tachycardia (VT), the rate is rapid and the rhythm is slightly irregular. There are no p waves because the impulse is generated in the ventricle. The QRS is widened because the depolarization does not go through the AV node nor the His-Purkinje system (**Figure 2.13**).

Nonsustained VT (NSVT) is defined as three or more consecutive QRS complexes of ventricular origin at a rate of at least 100 bpm, but not exceeding 30 consecutive beats or 10 seconds of consecutive beats. Sustained ventricular tachycardia occurs when these limits are exceeded.

This is a life-threatening arrhythmia. Follow ACLS protocol. Rapid defibrillation may be required if the patient is pulseless.

Torsades de Pointes

Torsades de pointes ("twisting around the point") is an ominous, polymorphic form of VT. The impulse is initiated in the ventricle, but the origin rotates throughout the ventricle. This is reflected on the EKG by a wide-complex tachycardia that rotates its axis as shown in **Figure 2.14**.

Torsades de pointes results from marked prolongation of the QT interval as may occur in the congenital Long QT syndrome or in patients on medications that prolong the QT interval. Class 1A, 1C, and 3 antiarrhythmics as well as medications that are metabolized through the CYP3A hepatic enzyme system have been implicated. A complete list of these medications can be found at **www.torsades.org**.

It is important to differentiate torsades de pointes from VT, because magnesium is required to treat torsades de pointes. When in doubt, consider administering 1 gram of magnesium during ACLS protocol.

Pearl

Look at the patient's medication list to see if they are on any QT prolonging drugs. QT prolongation may result in torsades de pointes.

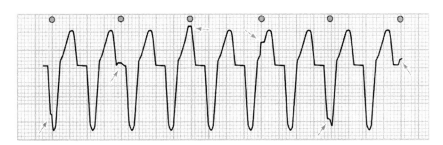

FIGURE 2.13   Ventricular Tachycardia

Source: Garcia, Tomas B., and Neil E. Holtz. 12-Lead ECG: The Art of Interpretation. Jones and Bartlett Publishers. 2001.

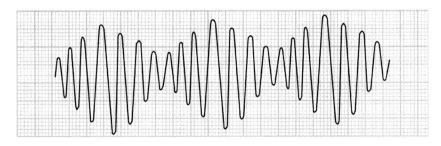

FIGURE 2.14   Torsades de Pointe

Source: Garcia, Tomas B., and Neil E. Holtz. 12-Lead ECG: The Art of Interpretation. Jones and Bartlett Publishers. 2001.

Ventricular Fibrillation

In ventricular fibrillation (VF), there are no regular QRS contractions; therefore, there is a bizarre pattern on the EKG as shown in **Figure 2.15**. VF is a life-threatening arrhythmia and is managed according to ACLS protocols. This involves immediate cardioversion followed by an IV antiarrhythmic such as amiodarone for 24–48 hours. Chronic management may include antiarrhythmic drug therapy or an ICD (implantable cardioverter-defibrillator).

Asystole

Asystole is the absence of cardiac electrical activity. It is sometimes referred to as cardiac standstill and is identified on the EKG as a "flatline." Follow ACLS protocol to manage asystole. Epinephrine, atropine, and transcutaneous pacing may be needed acutely with consideration of permanent pacemaker implantation.

Paced Rhythms

Pacer spikes are often hard to find. If you have a widened complex QRS, look carefully to see if pacemaker spikes are present. If you are not sure, ask the patient if they have had a pacemaker or palpate for the device just below the collarbone.

Quick and Easy Axis

Determining the axis is often made much more complicated than necessary. If attempting to identify the exact axis is overwhelming for you, simply note whether there is pathological right or left axis deviation.

If left axis deviation is present, then left ventricular hypertrophy (LVH), a left bundle branch block (LBBB), or a left anterior hemiblock may be present

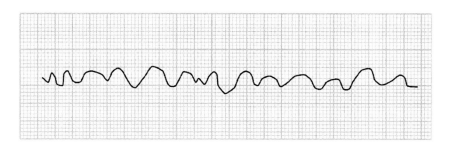

FIGURE 2.15   Ventricular Fibrillation

Source: Garcia, Tomas B., and Neil E. Holtz. 12-Lead ECG: The Art of Interpretation. Jones and Bartlett Publishers. 2001.

and should be sought. These abnormalities result in left axis deviation (LAD) and are often overlooked by clinicians who are looking for more overt abnormalities on the EKG such as ischemic changes or arrhythmias. Although it is less common, LAD may also be caused by mechanical rotation of the heart as may occur with ascites.

If right axis deviation (RAD) is noted on the EKG, look carefully to determine if there is a right bundle branch block, right ventricular hypertrophy, or a posterior hemiblock. RAD can also be caused by mechanical rotation. For example, chronic obstructive pulmonary disease (COPD) may cause the heart to be displaced toward the right due to hyperinflation of the lungs.

Bottom Line

Axis Deviation

Normal Axis	0 to 90 degrees (0 to negative 30 degrees is insignificant deviation, and is also considered normal)
Left axis deviation	More negative than −30 degreesRight axis deviation
Right axis deviation	More positive than 90 degrees

So how do you know if the axis is normal? Simply look in leads I and avF. If both of these QRS complexes reveal a predominantly positive deflection, which means that more of the waveform is located above the baseline, then the axis is normal. Yes, it really is that easy!

But what if one of these leads has a predominantly negative deflection? Simple again, if lead I is predominantly negative and avF is predominantly positive, then it is right axis deviation.

It gets just a little bit trickier if lead I is positive but avF is negative. In this case, left axis deviation is present, but up to negative 30 degrees of left axis deviation is considered normal. So if lead I is positive and lead avF is negative, look at lead II for confirmation. If lead II is upright, it is insignificant left axis deviation. If, however, lead II is negative, then a true left axis deviation exists.

Severe axis deviation is identified when both lead I and avF are negative.

Bottom Line

Axis	Lead I	Lead avF	Lead II
Normal	Up	Up	Not applicable
Right	Down	Up	Not applicable
Insignificant left	Up	Down	Up
Pathological left	Up	Down	Down

Intervals and Complexes

Once you have identified the rate and rhythm and decided whether left or right axis deviation is present, each interval and complex will need to be scrutinized for abnormalities.

The P Wave

The atria may stretch or dilate due to pressure or volume overload causing the p wave to appear abnormal.

P Mitrale

P mitrale is the EKG manifestation of left atrial enlargement, which may be caused by mitral stenosis (hence, the name "mitrale"). In mitral stenosis, the blood has difficulty passing from the left atrium to the left ventricle due to the stenotic mitral valve. This causes an increased volume of blood to remain in the atrium, resulting in atrial dilatation.

P mitrale is identified on the EKG by a broad, notched p wave in leads II and III. (It looks like an m, so think "the p looks like an m.") Additionally, the p waves will be biphasic in lead V1. This means that the p wave has an initial upward hump followed by a downward hump (**Figure 2.16**).

In western societies, p mitrale is most often attributed to hypertension.

Pearl

LAE (p mitrale) is often the first change that you will see on an EKG when hypertension has caused structural changes in the heart; use this as an opportunity to educate your patients about the importance of taking their blood pressure medicine regularly and adhering to lifestyle changes so that left ventricular hypertrophy and heart failure do not ensue.

P Pulmonale

P pulmonale is the EKG manifestation of right atrial enlargement, which may be caused by increased pulmonary pressure (hence, the name "pulmonale"). It is identified on the EKG by tall, peaked p waves in the inferior leads (II, III, and avF). You will also note a biphasic p wave in lead V1 (**Figure 2.17**).

The PR Interval

After assessing the p waves, measure the PR interval to ensure it is not too short or too long. The PR interval is normally 0.12–0.20 seconds, which is

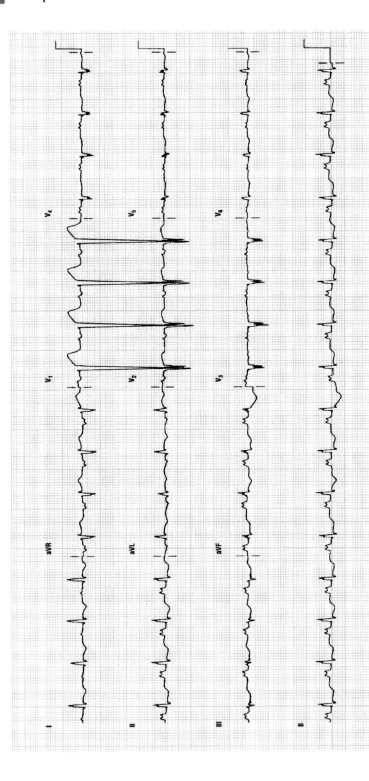

FIGURE 2.16 P mitrale

Source: Garcia, Tomas B., and Neil E. Holtz. 12-Lead ECG: The Art of Interpretation. Jones and Bartlett Publishers. 2001.

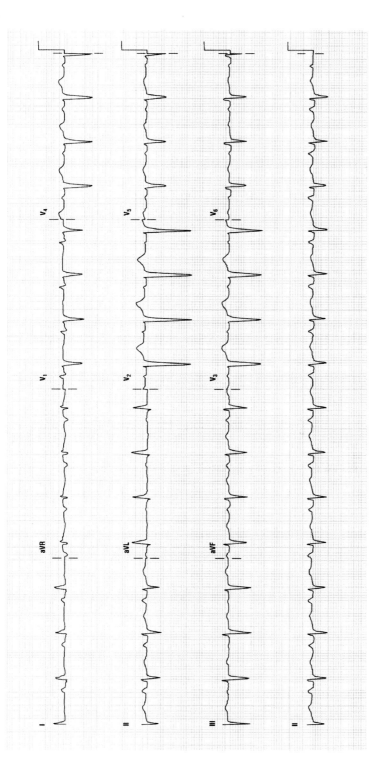

FIGURE 2.17 P pulmonale

Source: Garcia, Tomas B., and Neil E. Holtz. 12-Lead ECG: The Art of Interpretation. Jones and Bartlett Publishers. 2001.

Cardio Reality

During clinical skills check sheets, PA students are required to demonstrate proficiency in physical exam skills. While grading a student's performance, I noticed that he obtained a fairly elevated blood pressure on his fellow student who was acting as his patient. Over the next several months, the student monitored his blood pressure often and had instituted lifestyle changes.

When it came time for the EKG component of the curriculum, we learned that his father had suffered from an aortic dissection. Because HTN is the most significant risk factor for developing aortic dissection, I chose to perform the demonstration EKG on this student to see if he had any signs of hypertensive changes on his EKG. He had p mitrale, which indicated that he was already beginning to have structural changes related to elevated blood pressure. In light of his family history of aortic dissection and this EKG abnormality, I advised him to see a doctor. He chose a PA instead, and he was placed on antihypertensive medication. His blood pressure is now in the normal range and I hope that his early treatment will protect him from following in his father's medical footsteps. So, remember to look for—and act upon—the subtle clues that will help you protect your patients (and perhaps students) from developing future catastrophic heart disease.

represented by three to five small boxes on the EKG. PR prolongation may occur in first degree AV block while a short PR interval may occur in pre-excitation syndromes.

Bottom Line

PR prolonged	First degree AV Block
PR shortened	Preexcitation syndrome*

* Represents lack of delay in AV node such as with an accessory pathway. For example, Wolf Parkinson White (WPW)

Heart Block

Abnormalities of the PR interval may also be seen in heart block (AV block). First-degree heart block results from an increased delay in the AV node and is manifested as a prolonged PR interval (**Figure 2.18**).

Second-degree heart block occurs when some p waves do not conduct through the AV node at all. This results in some p waves not being followed by a QRS. There are two types of second-degree heart block.

In Mobitz Type 1 second-degree heart block (Wenckebach), the PR interval gradually lengthens until a QRS complex is dropped. The PR interval is, therefore, variable as shown in **Figure 2.19**.

Wenckebach occurs because the AV node gets fatigued. The first beat in the sequence is conducted quickly through to the ventricle. Then the AV node gets a little tired, so the next p wave takes a little longer to conduct, then a little longer, then the AV node is simply too tired to conduct at all. After dropping a QRS, the AV node is no longer tired and the cycle begins again. Wenckebach is not serious and does not require a pacemaker. You may see this rhythm in athletes who have good vagal tone.

Mobitz Type 2 second-degree heart block is more ominous than Type 1 because the QRS complexes drop out without warning. The PR interval remains constant and the rhythm may appear to be sinus when suddenly there is a p wave that is not followed by a QRS (as shown in **Figure 2.20**). This requires evaluation for a pacemaker.

In third-degree heart block (complete heart block), the AV node is completely blocked and there is no conduction from the atrium to the ventricle. The QRS complexes are generated independently from the ventricle. The p waves

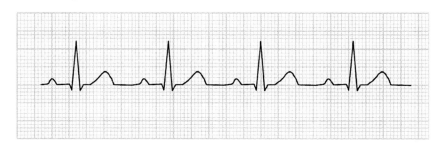

FIGURE 2.18   First Degree Heart Block

Source: Garcia, Tomas B., and Neil E. Holtz. 12-Lead ECG: The Art of Interpretation. Jones and Bartlett Publishers. 2001.

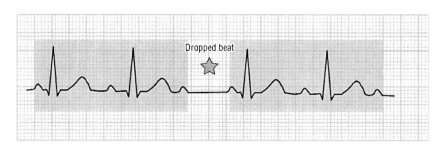

FIGURE 2.19   Mobitz Type I Second Degree Heart Block

Source: Garcia, Tomas B., and Neil E. Holtz. 12-Lead ECG: The Art of Interpretation. Jones and Bartlett Publishers. 2001.

are, therefore, completely dissociated from the QRS complexes. The PR interval will be variable as the atria are conducting at a different rate than the ventricles. If the ventricular impulse is generated fairly high up in the ventricle, then the ventricular rate may not be too slow and the QRS complex may even appear narrow. If the impulse is generated low in the ventricle, then the rate will be slower and the QRS complex will appear widened (**Figure 2.21**).

The QRS Complex

There are several things to analyze within the QRS complex. These include assessing the height and width of the complex, whether pathological Q waves are present, and whether the R wave progression is normal.

If the QRS appears wide, you should think of the following possibilities: a bundle branch block, a toxic conduction delay caused by drugs or hyperkalemia, a ventricular origin (such as PVCs or a paced rhythm), or a preexcitation syndrome such as Wolff-Parkinson-White.

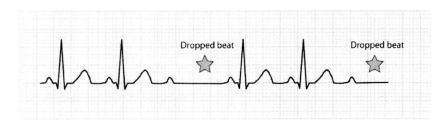

FIGURE 2.20   Mobitz Type II Second Degree Heart Block

Source: Garcia, Tomas B., and Neil E. Holtz. 12-Lead ECG: The Art of Interpretation. Jones and Bartlett Publishers. 2001.

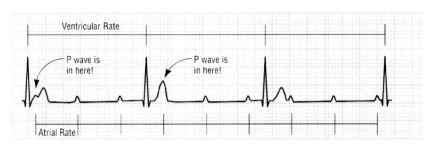

FIGURE 2.21   Third Degree Heart Block

Source: Garcia, Tomas B., and Neil E. Holtz. 12-Lead ECG: The Art of Interpretation. Jones and Bartlett Publishers. 2001.

Bottom Line		
Type of Block	PR interval	QRS complexes
1st Degree	Constant, prolonged	None dropped
2nd Degree, Type 1 (Wenckebach)	Variable, gradually lengthens	Some dropped, regularly
2nd Degree, Type 2	Constant	Some dropped, randomly
3rd Degree	Extremely variable	Completely dissociated

Bundle Branch Blocks

The width (or duration) of the QRS complex should be less than 0.10 seconds, which is two and a half small boxes on the EKG. A conduction system abnormality involving either the left or the right bundle exists if the width is greater than 0.12 seconds. A QRS duration between 0.10 and 0.12 seconds is considered an incomplete bundle branch block.

In a left bundle branch block (BBB), the QRS in Leads 1 and V6 are upright, wide, and notched (**Figure 2.22**). Because the left bundle splits in two, it is possible to have a left hemiblock if the left bundle is blocked after it splits into two. If the anterior fascicle is blocked, it is called a left anterior hemiblock (fascicular block). This presents as a large S wave (at least one small box deep and wide) in the inferior leads (II, III, and avF). It must be present in all three of the leads, not just one or two (**Figure 2.23**). If the posterior fascicle is blocked, which is much less common, there will be S waves in leads I and avL.

In a right BBB, the QRS in Leads 1 and V6 have a slurred s wave. For confirmation, you can look in leads V1 or V2 for "rabbit ears" (RSR′ or RR′) (**Figure 2.24**).

Left Ventricular Hypertrophy

Once the width of the QRS has been assessed, the height is evaluated to determine whether left ventricular hypertrophy (LVH) exists. LVH indicates increased voltage of the left ventricle and is common in hypertensive heart disease. Although there are several different criteria for determining the presence of LVH, two simple ways of determining increased voltage are as follows:

1. If the S wave in V1or V2 plus the R wave in V5 or V6 is greater than or equal to 35mm.
   LVH = S (V1or V2) + R (V5 or V6) ≥ 35
   Select the larger S wave and the larger R wave when choosing between V1 and V2 and when choosing between V5 and V6 for your calculations.

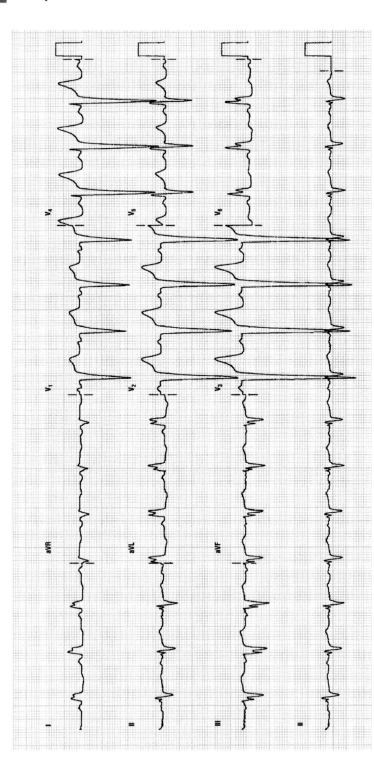

FIGURE 2.22 Left Bundle Branch Block

Source: Garcia, Tomas B., and Neil E. Holtz. 12-Lead ECG: The Art of Interpretation. Jones and Bartlett Publishers. 2001.

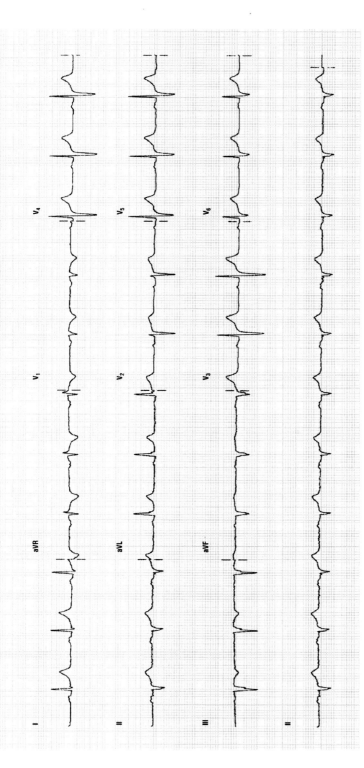

FIGURE 2.23 Left Anterior Fascicular Block

Source: Garcia, Tomas B., and Neil E. Holtz. 12-Lead ECG: The Art of Interpretation. Jones and Bartlett Publishers. 2001.

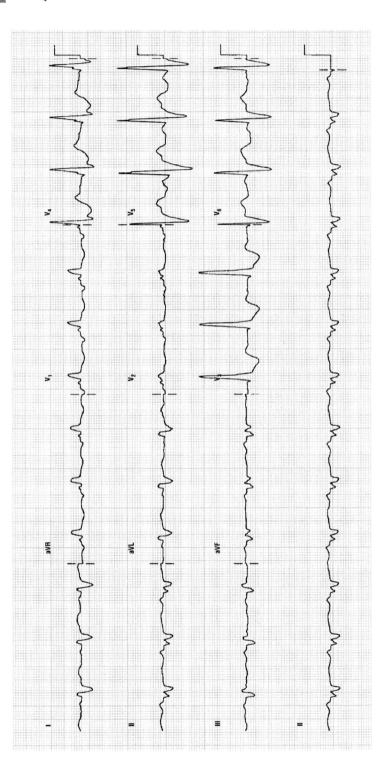

FIGURE 2.24 Right Bundle Branch Block

Source: Garcia, Tomas B., and Neil E. Holtz. 12-Lead ECG: The Art of Interpretation. Jones and Bartlett Publishers. 2001.

2. If the R wave in avL is greater than or equal to 11mm.
   If either of these voltage criteria are met, LVH exists (**Figure 2.25**).

It is important to identify LVH because it indicates that the ventricle has begun to thicken or
hypertrophy. If the disease process is allowed to
progress, heart failure, which has a very high
5-year mortality rate, may ensue. Therefore, hypertensive patients who have LVH on their EKG
need to be counseled strongly to maintain tighter
blood pressure control. It is also important to
identify LVH because it is often accompanied
by ST segment and t wave abnormalities (often
called a *strain pattern*) that can be easily mistaken for ischemia.

> **Pearl**
> Remember to look for
> LVH (also be sure to
> exclude a left BBB or
> a left hemiblock)
> whenever you have
> left axis deviation.

Right Ventricular Hypertrophy

When right axis deviation is observed, look carefully for right ventricular hypertrophy (RVH). If the R wave is greater than the S wave in leads V1 and/or
V2, the patient may have RVH. Unfortunately, this EKG pattern may also be
seen in a posterior MI or a right bundle branch block.

The ST Segment

Careful evaluation of the ST segment is important to identify ischemia or infarct patterns. However, ST segment abnormalities may be a result of other
pathology or may be a normal variant. In fact, ST segment elevation of up to
1 mm in the limb leads and up to 2 mm in the precordial leads may be normal.
You may notice ST segment depression in patients with LVH with a strain pattern or as a false positive. Digoxin causes a scooped appearing ST segment
depression as shown in **Figure 2.26**.

ST segment depression may be upsloping, horizontal, or downsloping. Upsloping ST depression is usually not significant. On the other hand, horizontal or downsloping ST segment depression is strongly indicative of ischemia.
(**Figure 2.27**).

ST segment elevation is the classic presentation of an acute myocardial
infarction. These elevations often appear like "tombstones" on the EKG.
Figure 2.28 shows classic ST elevation in leads V1 through V3 consistent with
an acute MI in the anteroseptal region. Other causes of ST elevation include
pericarditis and a ventricular aneurysm. If the ST segment elevation is a result of an infarct, the elevations should appear in anatomically contiguous

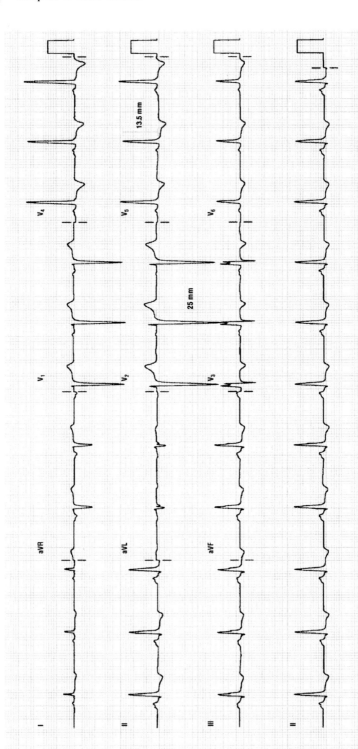

FIGURE 2.25 Left Ventricular Hypertrophy

Source: Garcia, Tomas B., and Neil E. Holtz. 12-Lead ECG: The Art of Interpretation. Jones and Bartlett Publishers. 2001.

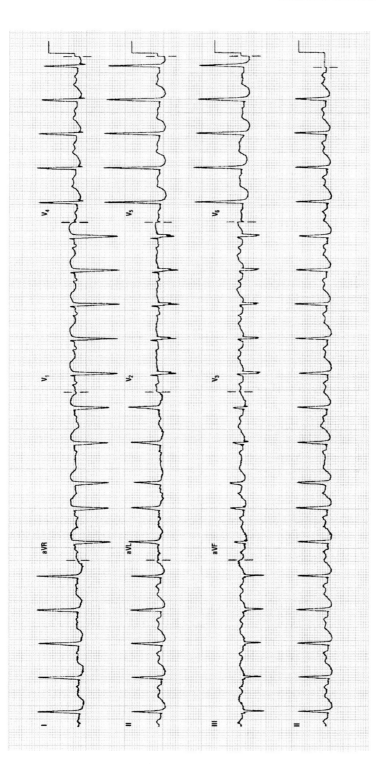

FIGURE 2.26 Scooped ST Depression Due to Digoxin Effect

Source: Garcia, Tomas B., and Neil E. Holtz. 12-Lead ECG: The Art of Interpretation. Jones and Bartlett Publishers. 2001.

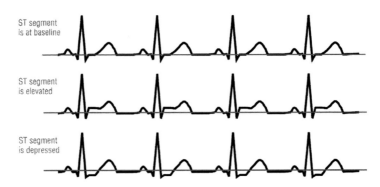

FIGURE 2.27 ST Segment Elevation and Depression

Source: Garcia, Tomas B., and Neil E. Holtz. 12-Lead ECG: The Art of Interpretation. Jones and Bartlett Publishers. 2001.

areas. For instance, an inferior MI should have abnormalities in all of the inferior leads: II, III, and avF. There should also be reciprocal changes, ST depression and/or T wave inversion, in other leads.

If ST elevation is due to pericarditis, then you will typically notice diffuse ST elevation with no reciprocal changes.

A ventricular aneurysm may occur after a myocardial infarction and is usually identified prior to discharge because the ST elevation does not normalize. If you suspect a ventricular aneurysm, request a copy of the EKG from the day of discharge. If the ST segments had returned to baseline and are now elevated again, you may have another infarct on your hands. If, however, the patient was discharged home with residual ST segment elevation, the patient may indeed have a ventricular aneurysm.

The T Wave

T waves may have variable appearances and t wave abnormalities are often nonspecific in terms of their diagnostic value. In hyperkalemia, you will note tall, peaked t waves. If the hyperkalemia is severe, the QRS widens until it looks like a sine wave.

In an early MI, the t waves appear peaked, like arrowheads. Flattened t waves are nonspecific. Inverted t waves may represent ischemia or a non-ST elevation MI (NSTEMI).

In patients with LVH, repolarization abnormalities caused by the hypertrophied ventricle may cause a strain pattern to appear on the EKG. A strain pattern may appear as concave downward ST depression and t wave inversion in the lateral precordial leads (V4–V6) with concave upward ST elevation in leads V1–V3 (**Figure 2.29**).

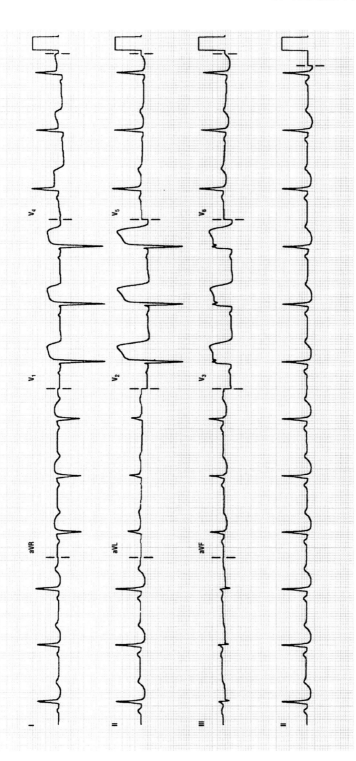

FIGURE 2.28 ST Elevation Due to Anteroseptal MI

Source: Garcia, Tomas B., and Neil E. Holtz. 12-Lead ECG: The Art of Interpretation. Jones and Bartlett Publishers. 2001.

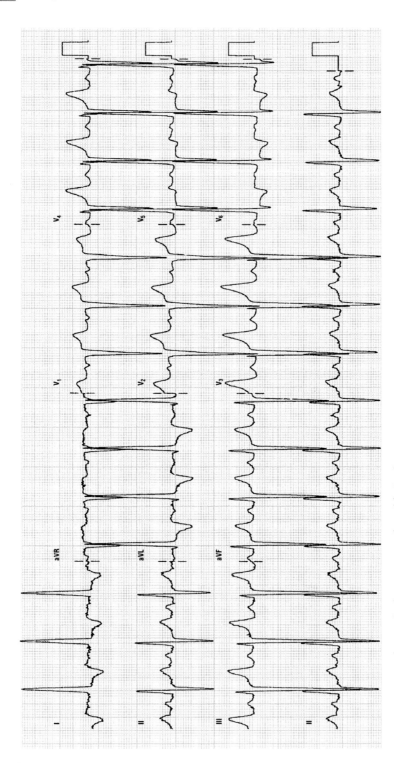

FIGURE 2.29 Left Ventricular Hypertrophy with Strain Pattern

Source: Garcia, Tomas B., and Neil E. Holtz. 12-Lead ECG: The Art of Interpretation. Jones and Bartlett Publishers. 2001.

The QT Interval

It is important to assess the QT interval because a prolonged QT may precipitate sudden death due to polymorphic ventricular tachycardia (torsades de pointes). The QT interval gets longer with a slower heart rate and vice versa. The QTc corrects for the heart rate and is normally less than or equal to 0.44 seconds. The formula for measuring the QTc involves a square root and so many try to avoid its use. Instead they use the following tricks for eyeballing the QT interval: Ensure that the QT interval is less than two large boxes. If it is not, then make sure that the QT interval is shorter than one-half of the R-R interval. If either of these criteria is met, then the QT interval is probably acceptable.

When an exact measurement is required, such as when monitoring antiarrhythmic medication, it is better to use the more exact formula. Such formulas can be downloaded from medical math-type programs onto a handheld device.

A prolonged QT interval may be congenital (as in the well-named "Long QT syndrome") or a result of certain medications. Hepatic elimination of medications occurs primarily by the cytochrome P450 (CYP450) system of enzymes. Concomitant use of medications that are metabolized by the same CYP450 isoenzymes can overload the system resulting in toxicity including prolongation of the QT interval. Some typical culprits include antiarrhythmics (remember all antiarrhythmics are inherently proarrhythmic), antihistamines, tricyclic antidepressants, antipsychotics, certain antibiotics, antifungals, antivirals, intestinal medications such as cisapride (Propulsid), anticonvulsants, and so forth.

Pearl

Tricks for Eyeballing a QT

Make sure that the QT interval is less than two large boxes. If it is not, then make sure that the QT interval is shorter than one-half of the R–R interval. If either of these criteria is met, then the QT interval is probably okay.

The U Wave

Although they are not always visible, a u wave may be seen after the t wave. U waves are more prominent with hypokalemia. The u wave may blend with the t wave making the t wave appear wider and, therefore, their presence is sometimes mistaken for a prolonged QT interval.

Bottom Line

What Lead Should I Look At?

Axis	I and avF. Confirm LAD in II.
LAE (p mitrale)	II and III (broad and notched). V1 (biphasic).
RAE (p pulmonale)	II and III (tall and peaked). V1 (biphasic).
BBB	I and v6 (upright and notched in LBBB; down with slurred s wave in RBBB).
Inferior MI or ischemia	II, III, and avF.
Lateral MI or ischemia	I, avL, V5 and V6.
Anterior MI or ischemia	Precordial leads V1–V4 (anteroseptal is V3–V4 and anterolateral is V5–V6).
Posterior MI	Leads V1 and V2 (appears opposite of other MIs, so a large R wave may represent a Pathological Q wave here).

Chapter 3

Stress-Free Stress Testing and Other Cardiac Studies

Introduction

Once the initial evaluation has been completed, additional cardiac studies may be necessary to complete the work-up. Some tools of the trade and what they are most commonly used to assess are shown here:

Exercise stress test	Ischemia, exercise tolerance
Nuclear stress test	Ischemia, Ejection fraction (with sestamibi, but not with thallium studies)
Cardiac catheterization	CAD, Ejection fraction
Echocardiogram	Ejection fraction, valvular disease, structural abnormalities
MUGA	Ejection fraction
Holter Monitor	Arrhythmias
30 Day Monitor	Arrhythmias
Cardiac CT or MRI	Ischemia, structural or congenital abnormalities

Exercise Stress Tests

In addition to evaluating symptomatic patients for underlying ischemia, stress tests are often ordered to determine the effectiveness of treatment, to assess a patient's functional capacity, for cardiovascular screening in high-risk occupations (i.e., firefighters, truck drivers), prior to initiating exercise in older patients, and in asymptomatic patients with a high risk of coronary disease.

Although exercise testing is generally safe, myocardial infarction and death have occurred. For this reason, clinical judgment is essential in deciding which patients should undergo testing and proper back-up supervision must be available by an appropriately trained physician. To decide whether stress testing is appropriate, assess the patient's symptoms, review medications, review past and current significant medical history, and determine usual level of physical activity.

During the physical examination, evaluate the patient's ability to walk and exercise and look for signs of acute or serious illnesses that may prevent the patient from adequately performing the test. Additionally, determine the weight limit for the particular camera and table you are using at your facility; morbidly obese patients may exceed these limits.

Pearl

Physician assistants, nurse practitioners, and registered nurses under the direct supervision of a physician, who should be available for emergencies, can perform exercise testing safely on appropriate patients.

Bottom Line

Prior to performing any stress test, assess the patient to ensure they are not acutely symptomatic. Assess vital signs to ensure no significant hypotension, hypertension, bradycardia, or tachycardia. Listen for the murmur of aortic stenosis to be certain it wasn't missed.

Patient Selection

Absolute contraindications to exercise stress testing include severe aortic stenosis and acute cardiovascular conditions such as a myocardial infarction within the past 48 hours, unstable angina, symptomatic uncontrolled cardiac arrhythmias, symptomatic uncontrolled heart failure, acute pulmonary embolus or pulmonary infarction, acute myocarditis or pericarditis, and acute aortic dissection.

Relative contraindications include left main coronary stenosis, moderate stenotic valvular heart disease, electrolyte abnormalities, severe arterial hypertension (systolic BP >200 or diastolic BP >110), tachyarrhythmias or bradyarrhythmias, hypertrophic cardiomyopathy and other forms of outflow tract obstruction, mental or physical impairment leading to inability to exercise adequately, and high-degree atrioventricular block.

Additional Imaging

Adding imaging to the standard EKG interpretation of an exercise stress test increases the sensitivity and specificity of the study and offers an additional means to determine whether ischemia is present.

> **Pearl**
>
> Ensure the nitropaste or nitroglycerine patch has been removed because this may interfere with the results of the study.

An imaging agent, whether a nuclear agent (radioactive tracer) or an echocardiogram, is a useful addition if you have a higher index of suspicion that someone's symptoms are ischemia related or if the patient has an abnormal baseline EKG that will interfere with the interpretation of the results. In patients who are unable to exercise, a pharmacological agent can be used as a stressor in lieu of exercise. Pharmacological studies always have an additional imaging modality because the EKG findings are nondiagnostic if no exercise is performed.

Because there is a high false-positive rate when performing an exercise treadmill test in women, imaging agents are often added to prevent the need for a follow-up study to exclude ischemia. A stress echocardiogram is often ordered in such cases.

Imaging Agents

A nuclear study is performed by injecting the imaging agent (tracer) into the bloodstream while a gamma camera views the amount that reaches the heart muscle. Areas of the heart that have good blood flow will absorb the tracer while areas that are necrotic or severely ischemic will not. The tracer is injected and pictures are taken during both rest and stress and the images are compared. The tracer is eliminated in the urine or stool within 24 hours. A metallic taste in the mouth is often reported as a side effect.

There are several nuclear imaging agents. Thallium is rarely used anymore because of a high false-positive rate resulting from attenuation artifacts, particularly in obese patients or those with large, pendulous breasts. Thallium may still be used in thin patients because it is less costly than newer agents.

Newer technetium (Tc) agents such as Tc99m sestamibi (Cardiolite) and Tc99m tetrofosmin have fewer attenuation defects allowing for better images. However, obese patients or women with large, pendulous breasts will have optimal images performed if a 2-day imaging protocol is performed rather than

Bottom Line
Choose sestamibi or tetrofosmin (depending on which is carried by the facility) unless cost is a significant factor. Avoid thallium if the patient is obese or has large breasts.

completing the study in 1-day. These newer agents also provide a measure of the ejection fraction (EF) while a thallium scan will not.

Dual isotope imaging uses thallium for the initial rest images followed by either sestamibi or tetrofosmin for the stress images. This protocol allows the study to be completed in less time, but exposes the patient to significantly higher doses of radiation. This protocol is helpful in determining myocardial viability (how much of the heart is functioning) after sustaining a prior MI or in severe heart failure.

Regardless of which imaging agent is chosen, patients should be fasting to improve the quality of images by reducing attenuation in the gut.

Pharmacological Studies

Exercise is the ideal method of stressing the heart; however, patients with decreased functional capacity or chronic debilitation are unlikely to be able to exercise adequately to perform a quality study and would be better suited to having a pharmacological study. Patients who are taking beta-blockers or other negative chronotropic agents will be unlikely to raise their heart rate adequately by exercising and should either hold their medication or be considered for a pharmacological study.

Younger patients with functional impairment due to injury, arthritis, orthopedic problems, peripheral neuropathy, myopathies, or peripheral vascular disease may need a pharmacological study if it is unlikely that they will be able to exercise to a level that will raise their heart rate sufficiently.

Pharmacological Stressors

When performing a nuclear study, all three of the commonly used stressors—adenosine, dipyridamole (Persantine), and dobutamine—have similar sensitivity and specificity for the diagnosis of coronary artery disease. However, if you are using echocardiography instead of myocardial perfusion imaging, dobutamine is more sensitive. In stress-imaging studies, patients with a left bundle branch block, permanent pacemaker, or WPW should have the study performed with a vasodilator rather than dobutamine.

Dipyridamole is a vasodilator that has been replaced in most institutions by its short-acting metabolite, adenosine, because of rapid reversal of side effects. Due to the long half-life of dipyridamole, it is prudent to reverse its effects with aminophylline at the conclusion of the study.

Most pharmacological stress tests can be ordered with adenosine as the stressor unless the patient has bronchospastic lung disease (i.e., COPD or asthma), hypotension, or heart block/bradycardia.

Adenosine and dipyridamole may cause bronchospasm. Some providers are comfortable using these agents in patients with known COPD or asthma as long as they have milder disease (i.e., have never been intubated or required steroids) and are not actively wheezing. With experience, you will develop your own comfort level.

The vasodilators adenosine and dipyridamole will lower blood pressure so avoid using them if the patient is already hypotensive. Adenosine blocks conduction through the AV node and often causes heart block during stress testing; therefore, it should not be used if the patient has significant heart block or bradycardia at baseline.

Caffeine and theophylline block the binding of adenosine and dipyridamole and cannot be ingested within 24 hours of the study. This includes caffeine-free coffee and soft drinks, which still have a small amount of caffeine. If caffeine has been ingested, postpone the study or convert the study to a dobutamine study.

Dobutamine can be used in patients with severe COPD or asthma, but should be avoided in patients with poorly controlled hypertension or unstable carotid disease. Exercise caution if the patient has significant ventricular ectopy.

Dobutamine is a catecholamine that is given with a goal of attaining a target heart rate. Once the maximum dose of dobutamine has been given, atropine can be used as an adjunct to raise the heart rate further. Do not give atropine to patients with glaucoma.

> **Bottom Line**
>
> Choose adenosine as a stressor if the patient cannot or should not exercise. If the patient has had caffeine or theophylline within 24 hours, has severe or acute exacerbation of COPD or asthma, or has a contraindication to vasodilators such as hypotension or heart block/bradycardia, then choose a dobutamine study instead. Just be sure that the patient does not have severe hypertension, significant ventricular ectopy or unstable carotid disease prior to ordering a dobutamine study. Avoid atropine in patients with glaucoma.

Performing a Stress Test

Exercise Treadmill

Prior to performing the study, the patient's target heart rate is calculated and an exercise protocol is selected. The target heart rate is usually 85% of the maximum predicted heart rate. To obtain this number, simply subtract the patient's age from the number 220, and then multiply this number by 0.85. This is the heart rate you are trying to achieve during the study. The Bruce protocol, which increases the incline and speed of the treadmill every 3 minutes, is one example of an exercise protocol. The modified Bruce protocol is often chosen for the elderly because it begins at a slower pace and advances more gradually.

If an imaging study is performed, the tracer should be injected when the patient is close to peak exercise. They will need to continue to exercise for an additional minute or two to complete the study. Never terminate the study because the target heart rate has been reached; the study should be continued until symptoms such as fatigue, dyspnea, angina, dizziness, ataxia, cyanosis, or pallor warrant termination. Additional indications for early termination of the study include:

- ST depression greater than 2 mm
- ST elevation greater than 1 mm in leads other than V1, aVR, or those that contain a pathological Q wave
- Sustained tachyarrhythmia
- Development of a widened QRS complex, which may be due to a left BBB or an intraventricular conduction delay (IVCD), but that cannot be distinguished from VT
- Drop in systolic BP of greater than 10 mmHg despite increased workload if other ischemic signs exist
- Patient request to terminate the study

The patient should have continuous EKG monitoring during the study and for at least 5 minutes into the recovery phase. Blood pressure and heart rate should be recorded at each stage of exercise (every 3 minutes), at peak exercise, and during recovery. The patient should be continuously monitored for the development of any symptoms.

Adenosine Stress Test

Adenosine is an alpha-receptor agonist that increases myocardial blood flow by coronary vasodilatation. Because it is nonselective, it also may cause AV block, peripheral vasodilatation, and bronchospasm. Side effects are short lived due to its extremely brief half-life of only 5 seconds.

Adenosine is administered via an infusion pump over 4–6 minutes at a dose of 140 μg/kg/min. The imaging agent is given after 3 minutes of the infusion.

Contraindications include hypotension, sick sinus syndrome, high-degree AV block, and bronchospasm. Profound sinus bradycardia (heart rate less than 40 bpm) is a relative contraindication. The medications dipyridamole (found in Aggrenox) and aminophylline should be discontinued 24 hours prior to the study. Caffeinated products should be discontinued 12 hours prior to the study.

Side effects are common with adenosine and include chest pain, dyspnea, flushing, dizziness, hypotension, and nausea.

Early termination of the study is indicated in the following circumstances:

- Severe hypotension (systolic BP less than 80 mmHg)
- Symptomatic, persistent high-grade heart block
- Severe chest pain associated with 2 mm or more of ST depression
- Signs of poor perfusion (pallor, cyanosis, cold skin)
- Technical difficulties with monitoring
- Patient request to terminate the study

Common complications include hypotension and significant heart block including asystole. Because of its short half-life, simply discontinuing the infusion of adenosine usually results in rapid improvement. In the case of hypotension, place the patient in the Trendelenburg position (or simply take the pillow out from under the head and pile pillows under the feet) and give IV fluid. In the case of asystole, follow ACLS protocol. Always have your crash cart available and know who to call for backup in the case of an emergency/code.

Dipyridamole Stress Test

Dipyridamole is a vasodilator that works by inhibiting the reuptake of adenosine. Its half-life is 40 to 80 minutes.

Contraindications are the same as with adenosine and include hypotension, sick sinus syndrome, high-degree AV block, and bronchospasm. Exercise caution in patients with hepatic dysfunction because dipyridamole is metabolized by the liver.

To perform the study, infuse at 0.56 mg/kg intravenously over 4 minutes and administer the radionucleotide at 7 to 9 minutes from initiation of the infusion.

Side effects are less common than with adenosine, but are longer lived. If you choose to reverse the effects of dipyridamole, give intravenous aminophylline (125–250 mg) to the patient at 12 minutes after you initiated the infusion. (You can give this as early as 9 minutes after initiation if the patient is extremely uncomfortable due to adverse effects of the agent).

If complications arise, administer aminophylline and utilize your ACLS protocols. Treat hypotension by placing the patient in the Trendelenberg position and administering IV fluids.

Dobutamine Stress Test

Dobutamine is a catecholamine that is primarily a beta 1 agonist. It causes increased chronotropy (heart rate) and increased inotropy (contractility), which results in increased oxygen demand similar to exercise. It is used principally for patients who cannot exercise or tolerate a vasodilator. Its half-life is 2 minutes.

Contraindications include a history of MI (within 7 days), unstable angina, history of ventricular arrhythmias, atrial arrhythmias with an uncontrolled ventricular response, severe aortic stenosis, hemodynamically significant left ventricular outflow tract (LVOT) obstruction, aortic aneurysm or dissection, and uncontrolled hypertension (blood pressure greater than 200/110). The infusion is initiated at 5 to 10 μg/kg/min and titrated every 3 minutes to a maximum dose of 40 μg/kg/min. The radionucleotide is injected at peak stress. Arm or leg exercise can be performed concomitantly to augment heart rate response by having the patient squeeze stress balls and/or repeatedly raise their legs off the table. The goal of the study is to reach 85% of maximum predicted heart rate. Atropine is often employed if these measures fail to achieve this goal. Remember not to use atropine if the patient has glaucoma. When the target heart rate has been reached or the maximum dosages of dobutamine and atropine have been given, the study has been completed.

Early termination of the study is indicated in the following circumstances:

- Systolic blood pressure exceeds 230 mmHg
- Diastolic blood pressure exceeds 130 mmHg
- Systolic BP drops below 80 mmHg
- Severe angina or other intolerable symptoms
- Significant ST segment depression (greater than 2 mm from baseline)
- Ventricular tachycardia (more than five beats)
- 2:1 or complete heart block

Side effects are common and include palpitations, chest pain, headache, flushing, dyspnea, and significant arrhythmias.

Sustained atrial fibrillation and ventricular tachyarrhythmias may occur, so be prepared. Fortunately, they are generally well tolerated and do not require treatment. Beta-blockers will reverse the effects of dobutamine and should be given first-line if needed (i.e., 0.5 mg/kg of IV esmolol over 1 minute or 5 mg of IV metoprolol).

Holding Medications

If the patient is undergoing a diagnostic study using a pharmacological stressor, beta-blockers, nitrates, and calcium channel blockers may alter the results and should be held. Hold beta-blockers for 48 hours prior to the study and hold calcium channel blockers and oral nitrates for 24 hours. If, however, the purpose of the study is to determine if the patient is on appropriate medical management or to follow-up after an intervention, then these medications should be continued.

Documenting Results

1. Provide a baseline EKG interpretation.
2. Record any chest pain, shortness of breath, or other pertinent symptoms.

3. Specify the reason for ending exercise if a treadmill study was performed; fatigue is the most common reason. (Don't stop an exercise stress test just because you have achieved the target heart rate.)

4. Note "target heart rate achieved" or "submaximal study" based on reaching the 85% of maximal heart rate goal. (This only applies to exercise or dobutamine studies.)

5. Note "normal BP response" or "hypertensive (or hypotensive) response."

6. Note any arrhythmias or ectopy and document their frequency and when they occurred (i.e., during peak exercise or in recovery).

7. Note whether ST elevation or depression was present and in which anatomical area. Remember that ST segments must remain below the baseline for at least 0.08 seconds (two small boxes) past the j point or it is a normal response to exercise.

8. If the study involves images or echocardiography, add: "Images/Echo report pending." This prevents others from misinterpreting the procedural note as the final report.

Interpretation of Nuclear Images

In a nuclear stress test, rest images and stress images are obtained and then compared. In a normal study, the radioactive tracer is evenly distributed throughout the heart muscle and no areas of abnormal tracer absorption are present during stress or rest images. In an abnormal study, areas of decreased uptake may indicate that some areas of heart muscle are not receiving adequate blood supply. If the absorption in these areas is normal at rest but reduced with stress, then ischemia is likely. This is often described as a reversible defect. If the absorption is decreased with both rest and stress, then an old infarct is likely. This is often described as a fixed defect.

Echocardiogram

An echocardiogram uses sound waves to image cardiac structures and evaluate blood flow. As the sound waves encounter structures with different densities, some of the ultrasound waves are reflected back to the transducer and recorded. A standard echocardiogram is performed through the chest wall, the transthoracic approach.

A two-dimensional echocardiography, which creates an image by passing an ultrasound beam across a 90-degree arc rapidly, is commonly used to assess cardiac size, structure, and function.

Doppler echocardiography allows assessment of both direction and speed of blood flow within the heart and great vessels. The motion of red blood cells changes the energy of the ultrasound waves; the transducer records this energy change. The magnitude of this change (Doppler shift) can be used to determine if the blood flow is normal or abnormal. This measurement can be converted to pressure allowing for the assessment of pressure gradients across valves or between chambers.

Color Doppler imaging allows visualization of blood flow through the heart by assigning a color to the red blood cells based on their speed and direction. Blood moving away from the transducer is represented in shades of blue and blood moving toward the transducer is represented in red. This color scheme is particularly useful in identifying valvular insufficiency and abnormal shunt flow between chambers.

Trans-Esophageal Echocardiogram

A trans-esophageal echocardiogram (TEE) is an echocardiogram that is performed by passing a gastroscope with an ultrasound crystal at its tip down the patient's esophagus. The close proximity of the esophagus to the heart provides a good view of the left atrium, mitral valve, and aorta.

A TEE is useful in diagnosing aortic dissection, endocarditis, prosthetic valve dysfunction, and left atrial masses. It is often performed to look for an atrial thrombus prior to a cardioversion.

Multiple-Gated Acquisition Scan

A multiple-gated acquisition scan (MUGA) is performed by tagging a radioactive isotope, Technetium 99, to red blood cells. The patient is then placed under a gamma camera, which detects the low-level radiation being given off by the Technetium-labeled red cells. Since the tagged red blood cells fill the cardiac chambers, the chambers are outlined and a moving image of the beating heart is produced.

The MUGA is used to measure the left ventricular ejection fraction (LVEF) more accurately than the echocardiogram. The MUGA is useful in evaluating the cardiotoxic effects of certain chemotherapeutic agents or to follow the progress of patients who require more accurate measurements of EF, as in patients who may need heart transplantation. The level of radiation to which a patient is exposed during a MUGA scan is in the same general range as the level of radiation received with a chest X-ray.

Tilt Table Test

A tilt table test is often used in the evaluation of syncope. It is particularly useful if the diagnosis of neurocardiogenic syncope is suspected. Do not perform this test if the patient is orthostatic at baseline.

Performing a Tilt Table Test

This test is conducted in a quiet room because any distractions may prevent the patient from having a syncopal spell. The patient is placed on the swinging bed and safety restraints are used to ensure they do not become injured. An IV is placed and an infusion pump is prepared in the event that IV fluids are required or isoproterenol is used during the study.

The patient is placed in a head-up tilt between 60 to 90 degrees for between 10 to 60 minutes. Some protocols administer isoproterenol or nitroglycerine if syncope doesn't occur during the initial period of tilting. Adding either of these agents will increase sensitivity but reduce specificity.

Isoproterenol is given with the intent of increasing the heart rate 25% over baseline. Patients should remain in the upright tilt for an additional 20 to 30 minutes after administration of isoproterenol. Isoproterenol should be avoided in patients with coronary artery disease because it may provoke life-threatening arrhythmias in this population.

Some protocols utilize nitroglycerine instead of isoproterenol. Nitroglycerine will decrease the venous return, which will cause a reduction of blood pressure. One would expect a compensatory increase in heart rate in normal patients. However, in neurocardiogenic syncope, the patient will develop bradycardia in conjunction with hypotension and then become syncopal.

Blood pressure, heart rate, and symptoms should be continuously monitored and recorded every few minutes. Be prepared for episodes of marked hypotension and bradycardia with possible asystole. Don't panic, just place the person in the Trendelenberg or supine position and administer fluids; the patient should respond very quickly.

A positive test occurs if the patient develops loss of postural tone or loss of consciousness with a drop in blood pressure (vasodepressor response) or heart rate (cardioinhibitory response).

Cardiac Catheterization

A cardiac catheterization is an invasive procedure in which catheters are introduced percutaneously to evaluate the coronary arteries. It allows for the direct measurement of intracardiac pressures as well as visualization of the coronary arteries, cardiac chambers, and great vessels. Filling pressures and the ejection fraction can also be obtained.

Cardiac catheterization is generally indicated when a cardiac abnormality is clinically suspected and requires confirmation. For example, in a patient with multiple cardiac risk factors who presents with classic anginal symptoms and EKG abnormalities or in a patient with an abnormal stress test. Cardiac catheterization often precedes some type of intervention, such as angioplasty, bypass surgery, or valvular surgery.

Cardiac catheterization is generally safe, but informed consent must be obtained. Discuss the risks, benefits, and alternatives and document in the patient's chart that this has been done and that the patient has agreed to proceed. The risk-to-benefit ratio of cardiac catheterization is favorable if the patient has symptoms that negatively impact his or her lifestyle or potentially fatal cardiac disease.

Patients should be advised of the following: "There is about a 1 in 1000 risk of death, heart attack, or stroke as well as about a 1 in 500 risk of arrhythmias or infection and a 1 in 100 risk of vascular damage, allergic reaction to the IV dye, or renal failure requiring dialysis." Consult with the physician performing the catheterization to ensure these percentages are compatible with his or her performance and then recite the risks every time a catheterization is considered. Note that infection is 10 times more common with the brachial artery approach than the femoral artery approach and there is risk of nerve damage with the brachial approach.

Patients who have a history of IV dye or shellfish allergy can be premedicated and still receive the dye. Ask the physician performing the procedure which protocol he or she prefers. Typically, the patient will receive a corticosteroid in conjunction with an H1 blocker and an H2 blocker. Additionally, the newer nonionic contrast agents have a cross-reactivity of less than 1% in patients with a history of a reaction to an older agent.

The risk of renal failure can be reduced by determining which patients are at risk and if clinically appropriate, delaying the catheterization or using low osmolal contrast, which has a lower dye load and is easier on the kidney. Additionally, in patients at high risk for renal failure, the catheterization can be done without doing a ventriculogram, which assesses ejection fraction. This reduces the amount of dye needed during the procedure. Be sure to alert the physician who will be performing the catheterization of the need to exercise renal caution. Keep the patient well hydrated; normal saline at 1 ml/kg/hr should be started 2 to 12 hours prior to the procedure and be continued for 6 to 12 hours after the procedure. Exercise caution in patients with heart failure who may be prone to volume overload. Acetylcysteine (Mucomist) 600 mg po BID can be prescribed on the day before and day of the procedure, although there is conflicting evidence of its utility.

Occasionally, the radial approach will be used to catheterize the patient. If this is planned, ensure that the patient has appropriate ulnar and collateral circulation to the hand by performing a modified Allen test. This way, if the radial artery is damaged, blood supply to the hand will remain intact and not result in loss of the hand. Simply elevate the patient's hand and have them make a fist while you occlude both the radial and ulnar artery. Once the blood has drained from the hand, lower it, have the patient open their fist, and release the ulnar artery while maintaining pressure on the radial artery. If color returns to the hand within 6 seconds, then the ulnar artery is supplying sufficient blood flow to the hand. An abnormal response is when it takes 10 or more seconds for the color to return to the hand.

Right-Sided Catheterization

In order to assess the pressures within the right atrium, right ventricle, and/or pulmonary artery, a right-heart catheterization is required. This is generally ordered as a "right and left heart cath" and assesses both sides of the heart. A right heart catheterization can determine the pressure gradients across the valves and is therefore useful in assessing patients prior to valvular surgery.

Cardiac Computed Tomography and Magnetic Resonance Imaging

Cardiac computed tomography (CT) and magnetic resonance imaging (MRI) are becoming widely available, but the utility of these tests is still being ironed out. It has been suggested that these modalities be considered for use in patients with ischemic symptoms or an abnormal stress test who refuse to undergo catheterization, to assess patency of bypass grafts that were poorly visualized during catheterization if the status of the graft is clinically important, and to evaluate coronary anomalies.

Cardiac CT images are adversely affected by motion artifact. For this reason patients are usually given a beta-blocker to slow their heart rate prior to the procedure. IV dye is used for this procedure; this study should be avoided if the patient is allergic to IV dye or is at high risk of developing contrast-induced nephropathy.

CT images will be poor in patients with a heart rate greater than 60–70 bpm or an irregular heart rhythm. Poor images also result if patients are unable to hold their breath for 15–20 seconds or if they have severe coronary calcification or cardiac stents in place (because metal or calcium causes artifact). Additionally, cardiac CT is not able to visualize small-caliber vessels well.

Cardiac MRI is preferred over cardiac CT in younger patients to avoid the significant amount of radiation exposure associated with cardiac CT. Additionally, cardiac MRI is preferred in patients who are unable to take beta-blockers or have contraindications to IV dye. Unfortunately, the cardiac MRI requires a skilled operator and is relatively contraindicated if metal or electrical devices such as pacemakers are present. However, stents are not contraindicated regardless of their type or time of implantation.

Cardiac MRI is useful in the evaluation of congenital anomalies such as right ventricular dysplasia and structural defects such as coronary artery aneurysms. Also, research is underway regarding their use as screening tools of asymptomatic patients or for follow-up of patients with known CAD. Significant advances are made with each new generation of cardiac MRI and CT and there is a need for direct visualization of the coronary artery lumen without the expense and risks that are associated with cardiac catheterization. For these reasons, the literature will likely support an increased role for cardiac MRI and CT in the near future.

Evaluating Heart Rhythm

Holter Monitor

The electrical activity of the heart is recorded for a 24- to 48-hour period while the patient keeps a diary of symptoms and activity. The rhythm strips are then analyzed, and any irregular heart activity is correlated with activity or symptoms.

Event Monitor

Event monitors (30-day monitors) are useful in patients who do not have symptoms every day. The monitor remains on the patient for 30 days, but is removed by the patient while bathing and the like . It only records episodes when the patient develops symptoms (dizziness, palpitations, CP, SOB, or syncope) and either presses a button or calls in to report the episode (depending on the brand used).

Implantable Loop Recorder

An implantable loop recorder is a heart monitor that is implanted under the skin where it can remain for many months. It is used to diagnose rhythm disturbances in patients who have very infrequent episodes of syncope or suspected heart arrhythmias. If the patient experiences symptoms, they see their cardiology provider who downloads the information and reviews the rhythm strips.

SECTION I RESOURCES

Akinpelu, D., and S. Reddy. 2003. *Treadmill and Pharmacologic Stress Testing.* Accessed from www.eMedicine.com. Retrieved June 26, 2006.

Baliga, Ragavendra, Anjana Siva, and Mark Noble. 2005. *Crash Course: Cardiology.* Philadelphia, PA: Elsevier Mosby.

Bickley, Lynn S. 2003. *Bates' Guide to Physical Examination and History Taking,* 8th ed. Philadelphia, PA: Lippincott Williams and Wilkins.

Carrozza, Joseph P., and Donald S. Baim. *Complications of Diagnostic Cardiac Catheterization.* Accessed from www.utdol.com. Retrieved September 28, 2006.

Crouch, Michael A., Lynn Limon, and Angela Cassano. "Clinical Relevance and Management of Drug-Related QT Interval Prolongation." *Pharmacotherapy* 23(7): 881–908.

DiPiro, Joseph P., Robert L. Talbert, Gary C. Yee, et al. 2005. *Pharmacotherapy: A Pathophysiologic Approach,* 6th Edition. New York, NY: McGraw Hill.

Dubin, Dale. 1991. *Rapid Interpretation of EKGs.* Tampa, FL: Cover Publishing Company.

Garcia, Tomas B., and Neil E. Holtz. 2001. *12-Lead ECG: The Art of Interpretation.* Sudbury, MA: Jones and Bartlett Publishers.

Henzlova, Milena, Manuel Cerqueira, John Mahmarian, and Siu-Sun Yao. "Stress Protocols and Tracers." *Journal of Nuclear Cardiology.* Vol 13: 6: 80–90.

Institute for Clinical Systems Improvement. 2004. *Cardiac Stress Test Supplement.* Bloomington, MN: Institute for Clinical Systems Improvement.

Olshansky, Brian. *Upright Tilt Table Testing in the Evaluation of Syncope.* Accessed from www.utdol.com. Retrieved August 21, 2006.

Rudnick, Michael R., James A. Tumlin, and Burton D. Rose. *Prevention of Radiocontrast Media-Induced Acute Renal Failure.* Accessed from www.utdol.com. Retrieved September 28, 2006.

Stein, Emanuel. 2000. *Rapid Analysis of Electrocardiograms: A Self-Study Program.* Philadelphia, PA: Lippincott Williams and Wilkins.

Velusamy, Muthu and Gary Heller. *Pharmacologic Stress Myocardial Perfusion Imaging: Testing Methodologies and Safety.* Accessed from www.utdol.com. Retrieved June 26, 2006.

Cardio Meds

The medications used in cardiology are frequently prescribed for more than one indication. To avoid repetition in subsequent chapters, many of the more commonly used cardiac medications will be discussed here. These include beta-blockers, calcium channel blockers (CCBs), nitrates, angiotensin converting enzyme inhibitors (ACE inhibitors), aldosterone receptor blockers (ARBs), aldosterone antagonists, diuretics, digoxin, aspirin, clopidogrel (Plavix), and antiarrhythmics.

Chapter 4

Beta-Blockers

BACK TO THE BASICS

Reviewing the role of the alpha- and beta-receptors will assist in understanding how beta-blockers function. The alpha-receptors are located in the arterioles and veins and are essentially responsible for peripheral vasoconstriction. The beta 1 receptors are located primarily in the heart; they increase heart rate (chronotropy), contractility (inotropy), and atrioventricular (AV) conduction (dromotropy). They also decrease AV node refractoriness. The beta 2 receptors are located primarily in bronchial and peripheral vascular smooth muscle. They bronchodilate and vasodilate as well as mobilize glucose and free fatty acids.

Bottom Line

Functions of Alpha and Beta Receptors

Alpha 1   Constrict peripheral arterioles and veins

Beta 1   Increase heart rate, contractility, and automaticity in the heart

Beta 2   Dilate bronchioles

Mechanism of Action

The beta-blockers block the "fight-or-flight" effects of catecholamines on the beta-receptors resulting in decreased heart rate, contractility, and automaticity. If the alpha 1 and beta 2 receptors are blocked along with the beta 1 receptors, bronchoconstriction and peripheral vascular dilatation may also occur.

Selecting a Beta-Blocker

Many beta-blockers are on the market and each has different characteristics. When choosing a beta-blocker, ensure that it has been proven beneficial for the condition(s) you are treating and consider the clinical implications of the chemical properties of the drug.

Indications

There are many conditions for which beta-blockers are prescribed, but only certain beta-blockers have been proven beneficial for some of these conditions. Try to choose a beta-blocker that has been proven to improve outcomes such as morbidity or mortality rates. The following is a list of indications accompanied by the specific beta-blocker(s) that have been proven beneficial for the condition:

1. Hypertension: All beta-blockers, except esmolol (Brevibloc), which is only adminstered intravenously, and sotalol (Betapace), are relatively equally effective.
2. Chronic atrial fibrillation: Sotalol (Betapace) is effective for maintaining sinus rhythm in patients with normal left ventricular function.
3. Post-MI: Atenolol (Tenormin) and metoprolol (Toprol XL, Lopressor) reduce early mortality post-MI and propranolol and timolol decrease late mortality.
4. Congestive heart failure: Bisoprolol (Zebeta), carvedilol (Coreg), and long-acting metoprolol (Toprol XL) have been shown to reduce mortality and hospitalization from heart failure.
5. Migraine prevention: Propranolol and timolol have proven efficacy, but metoprolol, nadolol, and atenolol have been shown to be effective as well.
6. Essential tremor: Propranolol has been proven beneficial.
7. Hypertrophic cardiomyopathy: Propranolol has been proven beneficial.
8. Pheochromocytoma: Propranolol has been proven beneficial.

Properties

When selecting a beta-blocker, it is important to understand some of the different chemical properties within this class of medications and their clinical significance. Beta-blockers differ regarding their cardioselectivity, lipid solubility, and whether they have intrinsic sympathomimetic activity.

Cardioselectivity

Cardioselective beta-blockers bind predominantly to cardiac beta 1 receptors, with much less affinity for the beta 2 receptors in the bronchi and peripheral blood vessels. This selectivity results in less bronchospasm when the cardioselective drugs are used at lower doses, but this benefit is lost at higher doses.

Cardioselective beta-blockers include atenolol (Tenormin), esmolol (Brevibloc), and metoprolol (Toprol XL, Lopressor).

Bottom Line

Beta 1 receptors predominate in the heart and beta 2 receptors predominate in the bronchi. As drug concentrations increase, binding becomes less selective even with cardioselective drugs. This causes a greater amount of adverse effects from the blockade of beta 2 receptors.

Intrinsic Sympathomimetic Activity

In addition to blocking the binding of catecholamines to the beta-receptor, beta-blockers with intrinsic sympathomimetic activity (ISA) also cause mild to moderate activation of the beta-receptor. The net result is less reduction in heart rate, less depression of atrioventricular (AV) conduction, and less negative inotropy than other beta-blockers. For this reason, beta-blockers with ISA tend to slow the heart rate less than other beta-blockers.

Avoid the use of beta-blockers with ISA in patients who are post-MI.

Acebutolol (Sectral), carteolol (Cartrol), penbutolol (Levatol), and pindolol (Visken) are all beta-blockers with ISA.

Lipid Solubility

Although not proven clinically, patients who suffer from fatigue or other CNS side effects may benefit from switching to a beta-blocker that has lower lipid solubility and therefore doesn't cross the blood-brain barrier as readily. CNS side effects include fatigue, depression, nightmares, insomnia, and hallucinations.

Carvedilol (Coreg), penbutolol (Levatol), and propranolol (Inderal) all have high-lipid solubility. Metoprolol (Toprol XL and Lopressor) and labetolol (Normodyne) have moderate-lipid solubility. Acebutolol (Sectral), atenolol

(Tenormin), bisoprolol (Zebeta), nadolol (Corgard) and sotalol (Betapace) have low-lipid solubility.

Pearl

Try not to become overwhelmed by all these lists of beta-blockers that do this and beta-blockers that do that. Keep it simple by selecting a few that you are comfortable with and stick with them. For instance, I choose to use predominantly metoprolol (Toprol XL) because it has been indicated for heart failure and hypertension and is cardioselective so I can expect to see fewer beta 2 mediated side effects. Additionally, it has been shown to lower mortality post-MI and it does not have ISA so it is safe to use in the post-MI patient. If these patients complain of central nervous system (CNS) side effects, I may consider switching them to atenolol because it is less likely to cross the blood-brain barrier. Although atenolol has not been shown to reduce mortality in heart failure, it has been shown to reduce mortality post-MI. Atenolol is also cardioselective and does not have ISA.

Contraindications and Precautions

Because they decrease the heart rate, beta-blockers are contraindicated in sinus bradycardia and high-degree AV block. Do not initiate during hypotension, acute decompensated heart failure, or cardiogenic shock.

Use caution in patients with bronchospastic lung disease (asthma or COPD); nonselective agents are generally contraindicated in patients with asthma and most patients with chronic obstructive lung disease.

Some patients with poor ventricular function rely on sympathetic stimulation to maintain their cardiac output; drugs that block the sympathetic response, such as beta-blockers, may worsen heart failure in these patients. For this reason, beta-blockers are usually initiated in patients with decompensated heart failure only after they are clinically stable.

The warning signs for hypoglycemia are mediated by the sympathetic nervous system and may not be noticeable once beta-blockers decrease sympathetic response. This could be devastating in brittle diabetics who are prone to hypoglycemic events. Beta-blockers can also delay the rate of recovery of the blood glucose concentration.

When initiating a beta-blocker, start with a low dose and increase gradually. Avoid abrupt discontinuation, which can lead to ischemia. Withdrawal syndrome may include accelerated angina, myocardial infarction, and even death; it can occur even in patients without previously known coronary disease.

Choose a calcium channel blocker and/or nitrate in patients with coronary artery spasm because beta-blockers may worsen this disorder.

Adverse Reactions

- Sinus bradycardia, sinus arrest, or AV block may occur due to negative chronotropy.
- Bronchospasm or bronchoconstriction may occur due to beta 2-receptor blockade.
- Fatigue may be due to the reduction in cardiac output or to direct effects on the central nervous system and may improve after a few weeks of therapy.
- Depression, insomnia, and delirium may also occur.
- Sexual disturbances may result.
- Severe peripheral vascular disease or Raynaud's phenomenon can be worsened with nonselective agents.
- Hepatic toxicity has been associated with labetalol.

Drug Interactions

Other drugs that depress myocardial function, such as calcium channel blockers and antiarrhythmic agents, may have added deleterious effects when used in combination with a beta-blocker.

Miscellaneous

Esmolol (Brevibloc) has a short half-life that enables IV use with the ability to reverse adverse reactions within 30 minutes of discontinuing the infusion. It is often used to control the heart rate in atrial arrhythmias after cardiac surgery.

In the event of an overdose of a beta-blocker, bradycardia, hypotension, low cardiac output, cardiac failure, and cardiogenic shock may occur. Bronchospasm, respiratory depression, mental status changes, convulsions, and coma may also occur. The myocardium in severe intoxications may become relatively refractory to pharmacologic and electrical stimulation resulting in asystolic death. Glucagon is used in the management of beta-blocker overdose.

In addition to hypotension and bradycardia, patients with sotalol intoxication may have significantly prolonged corrected QT intervals and severe ventricular tachyarrhythmias. These patients should be managed with intensive care including continuous cardiac monitoring and ventilatory support.

Beta-blockers have also been associated with the development of antinuclear antibodies, but rheumatic symptoms are infrequent. ANA titers and symptoms (if present) should resolve after the cessation of therapy.

Chapter 5

Calcium Channel Blockers

Mechanism of Action

Calcium channel blockers (CCBs) block the influx of calcium into the cells of the myocardium and the vasculature. Lower levels of calcium within these cells result in less stimulation and, therefore, less contraction. Less contraction within the myocardium reduces myocardial contractility, automaticity, and conduction velocity. Less contraction within the vasculature leads to dilatation of the blood vessels leading to decreased total peripheral resistance.

Selecting a CCB

CCBs are classified as either dihydropyridines or nondihydropyridines based on whether they bind predominately to the receptors in the myocardium or the receptors in the vasculature. Dihydropyridines bind primarily to the vasculature receptors and are potent vasodilators. They have little effect on myocardial contractility, impulse formation, or conduction velocity. Amlodipine (Norvasc), nifedipine (Procardia, Adalat), isradipine (DynaCirc), felodipine (Plendil), nicardipine (Cardene), and nisoldipine (Sular) are all examples of dihydropyridines.

The nondihydropyridines bind preferentially to the myocardium, reducing contractility, automaticity, and AV nodal conduction. The nondihydropyridines are easier to remember because there are only two of them, verapamil (Calan, Verelan) and diltiazem (Cardizem, Dilacor, Tiazac).

Indications

All of the dihydropyridines are indicated for management of hypertension but only amlodipine, nicardipine, and long-acting nifedipine are indicated in angina pectoris due to coronary spasm and chronic stable angina.

Diltiazem is indicated in angina pectoris due to coronary spasm, chronic stable angina, and hypertension. Verapamil is indicated for all of these conditions as well as in unstable angina and as adjunct therapy in obstructive hypertrophic cardiomyopathy.

Diltiazem and verapamil are indicated to control the ventricular rate in atrial flutter and atrial fibrillation, but should not be used if an underlying accessory bypass tract exists as in Wolff-Parkinson-White syndrome. They may also be used to convert paroxysmal supraventricular tachycardia to sinus rhythm if vagal maneuvers have failed.

Contraindications and Precautions

All CCBs are contraindicated in severe hypotension, cardiogenic shock, bradycardia, second- or third-degree AV block, and sick sinus syndrome. They are also contraindicated in atrial flutter or atrial fibrillation associated with an accessory bypass tract as in Wolff-Parkinson-White syndrome.

Dihydropyridines should be avoided in patients with severe aortic stenosis because vasodilatation results in reduction of preload and adequate diastolic filling is essential in these patients.

The nondihydropyridines are contraindicated in acute myocardial infarction, severe left ventricular dysfunction, and if pulmonary congestion is noted on chest radiography. Post-MI patients should generally avoid the use of CCBs, although a dihydropyridine may be considered if a compelling indication exists.

Exercise caution with CCBs in patients with underlying heart failure or severe hepatic impairment.

Adverse Reactions

Although the following list is not exhaustive, it includes some of the more common or serious adverse reactions associated with the CCBs.

Dihydropyridines

- Because they are potent vasodilators, edema is the most common side effect of the dihydropyridines.

- The other side effects of vasodilatation, which include flushing and headache, are less common in long-acting preparations.
- Hypotension
- Smooth muscle relaxation within the vasculature may result in reflex sympathetic activity causing tachycardia and increased cardiac output with the use of dihydropyridines.
- Isradipine and nifedipine are associated with more adverse reactions than other CCBs.

Nondihydropyridines

- Hypotension
- Bradycardia, AV block, or other arrhythmias
- Heart failure
- Constipation
- Flushing, headache, or edema due to vasodilatation. These side effects are more prominent with the dihydropyridines.
- Dizziness
- Verapamil may also cause depression.

Drug Interactions

The CCBs have many drug interactions because of the way they are metabolized through the hepatic cytochrome P450 system. Check a digoxin level and consider reducing the dose of digoxin when you add a CCB, particularly when adding a nondihydropyridine.

Exercise caution if using concomitantly with beta-blockers because heart failure, arrhythmias, hypotension, or conduction disturbances may result.

Avoid the long-term use of short-acting CCBs because they have been shown to worsen mortality in some patients.

Bottom Line

CCBs are both vasodilators and negative inotropes. Dihydropyridines are strong vasodilators whereas the nondihydropyridines are negative inotropes and negative chronotropes.

Chapter 6

Nitrates

Mechanism of Action

Nitrates such as nitroglycerine are converted to nitrous oxide (endothelium-derived relaxing factor), which relaxes the smooth muscle of the vasculature resulting in vasodilation. Vasodilation of the coronary arteries improves blood flow to ischemic areas of the heart. Vasodilatation of the peripheral veins reduces preload, thereby reducing myocardial oxygen demand. Both of these effects result in improvement of anginal symptoms.

Indications

Nitrates are indicated for the treatment of acute myocardial infarction, unstable angina, hypertension, congestive heart failure, and suspected ischemic chest pain.

Contraindications and Precautions

Right ventricular infarctions, which may occur in an inferior MI, often result in a stiff right ventricle that relies on sufficient preload to fill. Patients with aortic stenosis and hypertrophic obstructive cardiomyopathy also rely on sufficient preload. In these circumstances, use nitroglycerine with caution.

Use cautiously if hypotension or volume depletion is present and avoid abrupt discontinuation in chronic use; instead, reduce the dose gradually.

Adverse Reactions

- Headache and flushing are commonly reported
- Dizziness/syncope
- Weakness
- Palpitations/tachycardia
- Rash

Drug Interactions

Concomitant use of nitrates with the phosphodiesterase inhibitors sildenafil (Viagra), tadalafil (Cialis), and vardenafil (Levitra) is contraindicated. This combination can result in profound hypotension and, therefore, worsening ischemia.

Miscellaneous

Tell patients to sit or lie down when taking nitroglycerine to avoid syncope due to orthostasis.

Advise patient to call 911 if anginal symptoms are not relieved after the first nitroglycerine sublingual tablet. They may take two additional doses five minutes apart while a waiting Emergency Medical Services or while proceeding immediately to the ER.

Also, advise the patient to keep nitroglycerine away from heat sources (for instance, do not leave it in the car or a back pocket on hot days) and to be sure that they keep an eye on the expiration date. If a patient requires nitroglycerine sublingual but uses it infrequently, consider nitroglycerine spray. The spray is more costly initially but will not expire as quickly.

Tachyphylaxis may occur with nitrates. This means that nitrates may begin to lose their effectiveness over time, resulting in the need for escalating doses. This can be avoided by ensuring that patients have a nitrate-free interval of 8 to 10 hours daily. When prescribing nitropaste or a nitropatch, have it removed from 12 am to 8 am daily. (Write this in the orders.) When prescribing a twice-daily oral preparation (isosorbide dinitrate), tell your patient to take the medication at 8 am and 2 pm. The once-daily preparation (isosorbide mononitrate or Imdur) is designed to offer a nitrate-free interval. Because IV nitroglycerine is only utilized for short periods of time and is used for acutely ill patients who cannot afford to have the medication held, do not worry about a nitrate-free interval when ordering IV nitroglycerine.

Chapter 7

Renin-Angiotensin-Aldosterone Inhibitors

BACK TO THE BASICS

The kidney was designed to function as a filter. Each functioning unit (or fil-ter) within the kidney is called a *nephron,* and there are over one million nephrons in the kidney. Each nephron is made up of a glomerulus, which is where filtration occurs. A collection of tubes collect the waste products that are filtered out of the glomerulus and transport the waste into the ureters to exit the body as urine.

To allow the blood to filter out its waste products, the blood must pass through the nephron. Each nephron has an afferent arteriole leading the unfiltered blood into the glomerulus (where filtration occurs) and an efferent arteriole leading the filtered blood back to the bloodstream.

The kidney was designed with this unique arteriole-to-arteriole circulation to help regulate the pressure within the kidney. Arteries and arterioles have a muscular layer that allow for vasoconstriction, whereas veins and venules do not. The kidney's circulation was designed to have arteriole to arteriole rather than the standard artery to capillary to vein design in order to allow both the afferent arteriole and the efferent arteriole to constrict. The afferent

(continues)

BACK TO THE BASICS (continued)

---

arteriole needs to constrict to limit the blood pressure entering the kidney because the systemic blood pressure is twice as high as the pressure at which the glomerulus operates. This higher systemic pressure could destroy the delicate glomerulus. The efferent arteriole needs to be able to constrict in order to preserve the pressure needed for the glomerulus to function properly if the pressure within the glomerulus falls too low. This may occur in dehydration or excessive diuretic use (prerenal azotemia).

This intricate system of afferent and efferent vasoconstriction is mediated by the renin-angiotensin-aldosterone system. Renin is secreted by the kidney in response to glomerular hypoperfusion, reduced sodium, or in response to sympathetic nervous system stimulation. Renin is important in the formation of angiotensin II, which is both a potent vasoconstrictor and a stimulator of aldosterone. Angiotensin II constricts the efferent arteriole to help counteract the decreased blood volume in the kidney. Aldosterone's job is to retain sodium and water, which increases fluid volume, thereby increasing preload, thereby increasing cardiac output, and increasing the blood pressure.

Medications that inhibit the renin-angiotensin-aldosterone system include angiotensin-converting enzyme (ACE) inhibitors, angiotensin receptor blockers (ARBs), and aldosterone antagonists.

Angiotensin-Converting Enzyme Inhibitors

Mechanism of Action

ACE inhibitors block the conversion of angiotensin I to angiotensin II and block the breakdown of bradykinin, which is responsible for the cough that is frequently seen in patients taking ACE inhibitors. Essentially the ACE inhibitors reduce afterload by dilating the arterial circulation.

Selecting an ACE Inhibitor

The following ACE inhibitors have been shown to reduce morbidity and mortality in post-MI patients or those with heart failure: Captopril (Capoten), enalapril (Vasotec), lisinopril (Zestril or Prinivil), perindopril (Aceon), ramipril (Altace), and trandolapril (Mavik). It is unclear whether these benefits are a class effect shared by all ACE inhibitors.

Indications

ACE inhibitors are often used to manage hypertension, especially if the following compelling indications are present: heart failure, post-MI, diabetes mellitus, patients at high risk for coronary disease, prevention of recurrent stroke, and chronic kidney disease. In fact, the ACE inhibitors are the only hypertensive class that is recommended by the *7th Report of the Joint National Committee on Prevention, Detection, Evaluation, and Treatment of High Blood Pressure (JNC7)* for all six compelling indications identified in their report. When clinical trials have proven a reduction in morbidity and mortality with the use of a specific antihypertensive class to treat a hypertensive patient with an additional medical problem, that medical problem is described as a compelling indication for the use of that drug class.

Because ACE inhibitors have been shown to reduce morbidity and mortality in patients with heart failure as well as decrease progression of chronic kidney disease, all patients with these conditions should be placed on an ACE inhibitor unless it is contraindicated.

Contraindications and Precautions

ACE inhibitors are contraindicated in pregnancy and are especially detrimental to the fetus during the second and third trimester.

Although ACE inhibitors are renal-protective and therefore commonly used in patients with mild renal insufficiency, their use should be avoided in patients with creatinine levels greater than 3 mg per dL. Exercise caution if the patient has a potassium level greater than 5.5 mmol per liter or blood pressure less than 80 mmHg.

Avoid use in patients with bilateral renal artery stenosis or if patients have had previous life-threatening experiences such as angioedema or anuric renal failure due to ACE inhibitors.

Fluid retention can blunt the effects of ACE inhibitors and dehydration can increase the adverse effects of ACE inhibitors.

Avoid abrupt discontinuation in patients with heart failure because clinical decompensation may result.

Adverse Reactions

ACE inhibitors are very well tolerated in most patients, however, the following adverse reactions may occur:

- A dry cough may occur in up to 20% of patients. Consider switching patients to an ARB if patients develop this cough.

- Angioedema is a rare but life-threatening occurrence; if it occurs, the patient must avoid all ACE inhibitors and possibly ARBs because there may be cross-reactivity.
- Hyperkalemia may occur with the use of ACE inhibitors. Use caution in patients with renal insufficiency because renal impairment also results in hyperkalemia. Patients who are taking ACE inhibitors concomitantly with diuretics may not need potassium replacement. Be particularly cautious with patients on potassium-sparing diuretics.
- Neutropenia and agranulocytosis are rare but serious side effects.
- Glomerulonephritis and acute renal failure may occur rarely.

Pearl

The following mnemonic may assist you in remembering the adverse reactions associated with ACE inhibitors: **CAPTOPRIL** = **C**ough, **A**ngioedema, **P**roteinuria, **T**aste changes, **O**rthostatic hypotension (or just hypotension), **P**regnancy problems (fetal renal damage and increased fetal mortality if used during the second or third trimester), **R**ash, **I**ncreased renin, **L**ower angiotensin II and **L**ytes (stands for the electrolyte abnormality of hyperkalemia).

Drug Interactions

ACE inhibitors can increase lithium levels.

Hyperkalemia is more likely if ACE inhibitors are used concomitantly with aldosterone antagonists, potassium-sparing diuretics, ARBs, or potassium supplements.

Miscellaneous

Pearl

If a patient develops worse blood pressure control when an ACE inhibitor is initiated, consider the possibility of underlying renal artery stenosis.

ACE inhibitors may cause orthostatic hypotension, particularly in the elderly or volume-depleted: "Start low and go slow." Use low doses (half the usual starting dose) in these patients and titrate at 6-week rather than 2-week intervals.

It is more effective to add a diuretic to the regimen than to titrate the dose of an ACE inhibitor to achieve better antihypertensive control.

Check blood pressure, renal function, and potassium levels 1 to 2 weeks after initiation and then periodically. Clinical benefit in heart failure may take several weeks or months to become apparent.

ACE inhibitors are less effective antihypertensives in patients who are likely to have salt-sensitive hypertension (as in African Americans).

Angiotensin Receptor Blockers

Mechanism of Action

Angiotensin receptor blockers (ARBs) are similar to ACE inhibitors in that they also block the renin-angiotensin-aldosterone system. However, ARBs do not block the breakdown of bradykinin and therefore have the advantage of not causing the cough associated with ACE inhibitors.

Selecting an ARB

Although all ARBs are effective in lowering blood pressure, the following are true once-daily medications: Valsartan (Diovan), irbesartan (Avapro), olmesartan (Benicar), and telmisartan (Micardis). Because they have the shortest half-lives, losartan (Cozaar), candesartan (Atacand), and eprosartan (Teveten) may need to be dosed twice daily to achieve sustained blood pressure lowering.

Indications

ARBs have been shown to reduce progression of target-organ damage in hypertensive patients. Compelling indications for the use of ARBs in the hypertensive patient include chronic kidney disease, heart failure, and diabetes mellitus. ARBS have also been shown to significantly reduce the progression to nephropathy in patients with type 2 diabetes.

ARBs are often used in patients who are intolerant of an ACEI. ARBs are a relatively new class of antihypertensive and are generally more expensive than the ACE inhibitors. As more data reveals the merits of this class and as generic varieties become available, they will likely be viewed as first-line therapy for certain indications.

Contraindications and Precautions

The ARBs are contraindicated in pregnancy and are less effective in patients with salt-sensitive hypertension.

Patients who have had angioedema with ACE inhibitors may also have angioedema with the ARBs.

Adverse Effects

ARBs are extremely well tolerated, however, the following adverse effects may be seen:

- Hypotension
- Hyperkalemia
- Worsening renal function
- Angioedema may occur, but is less common than with ACE inhibitors
- Diarrhea
- Metallic taste
- Cough may occur, but is less common than with ACE inhibitors

Drug Interactions

ARBs may increase levels of lithium leading to potential toxicity.

Potassium supplements, salt substitutes (which often contain potassium), or other drugs that increase potassium may result in excessive blood potassium levels when used concomitantly with ARBs.

Miscellaneous

Check blood pressure, renal function, and potassium levels 1 to 2 weeks after initiation and then periodically.

It is more effective to add a diuretic to the regimen than to titrate the dose of an ARB to achieve better antihypertensive control.

Aldosterone Antagonists

Mechanism of Action

Aldosterone antagonists function at the mineralocorticoid receptor where they interfere with sodium and potassium exchange in the distal tubule. They essentially retain potassium while inhibiting resorption of sodium. This results in increased excretion of sodium and water.

Selecting an Aldosterone Antagonist

Spironolactone (Aldactone) and eplerenone (Inspra) are the only aldosterone antagonists currently available in the United States.

Indications

Aldosterone antagonists have been proven effective in reducing morbidity and mortality as part of the medical regimen in symptomatic heart failure and post-MI patients. These conditions are considered compelling indications for the use of an aldosterone antagonist in the hypertensive patient. Aldosterone antagonists are not, however, primary agents for the treatment of hypertension.

Contraindications and Precautions

Eplerenone is a very selective aldosterone antagonist and has a greater propensity to cause hyperkalemia. For this reason, eplerenone is contraindicated in patients with impaired renal function or type 2 diabetes with proteinuria. (Declining renal function in these patients increases their chances of developing hyperkalemia.) Serum potassium must be lower than 5.0 mEq/dL and creatinine less than 2.0 to 2.5 mg/dL.

Adverse Reactions

- Hyperkalemia
- Renal impairment
- Gynecomastia, impotence, and benign prostatic hyperplasia may occur with spironolactone, but are rarely seen in patients taking eplerenone.

Drug Interactions

Avoid nonsteroidal anti-inflammatory agents (NSAIDs) and cyclooxygenase inhibitors (COX 2 inhibitors) that may worsen renal function and increase the risk of hyperkalemia. Other medications that inhibit the CYP3A4 hepatic isoenzyme may significantly increase levels of eplerenone.

Chapter 8

Diuretics

Mechanism of Action

Several subclasses of diuretics are commonly employed for cardiac indications: the carbonic anhydrase inhibitors, loops, thiazides, and potassium-sparing agents, which include the aldosterone antagonists. Each segment of the nephron has a specific function and each subclass of diuretic functions at different locations along the nephron.

The proximal tubule is where organic solutes such as sodium bicarbonate and sodium chloride are reabsorbed. Also, 60% of water is reabsorbed from the kidney tubules into the bloodstream at this location. The carbonic anhydrase inhibitors block the reabsorption of sodium bicarbonate in the proximal tubule.

The loop diuretics function at the loop of Henle by blocking the reabsorption of sodium chloride; they also decrease the reabsorption of calcium and magnesium.

The distal tubule is the major area where potassium is regulated; this site is also where aldosterone functions to promote the reabsorption of sodium and water in an effort to increase blood volume. Potassium-sparing diuretics prevent aldosterone from functioning at the distal tubule either by blocking its receptors (spironolactone, eplerenone) or by interfering with the reabsorption of both sodium and potassium (triamterene and amiloride). The thiazides also work at the distal convoluted tubule to block the reabsorption of sodium chloride while increasing calcium reabsorption.

Selecting a Diuretic

Carbonic anhydrase inhibitors such as acetazolamide (Diamox) are rarely used today. Loop diuretics include furosemide (Lasix), bumetanide (Bumex), torsemide (Demadex), and ethacrynic acid (Edecrin). There are many thiazide diuretics; the more commonly used agents include hydrochlorothiazide (generic HCTZ, Microzide, Hydrodiuril), chlorthalidone (Thalitone), chlorothiazide (Diuril) and metolazone (Zaroxolyn).

Potassium-sparing diuretics include triamterene (Dyrenium), amiloride (Midamor), and the aldosterone antagonists spironolactone (Aldactone) and eplerenone (Inspra). Potassium-sparing diuretics are also packaged along with the thiazide diuretic HCTZ in the following poly-pills: Aldactazide (spironolactone plus HCTZ), Dyazide and Maxzide (triamterene plus HCTZ in different dosages), and Moduretic (amiloride plus HCTZ).

Indications

Loop diuretics are indicated in the treatment of edema as in congestive heart failure, acute pulmonary edema, or renal failure. They are also indicated in hypertension and hypercalcemia.

Thiazides are indicated in hypertension and mild heart failure. In severe, resistant edema, they can be used concomitantly with the more potent loop diuretics; metolazone (Zaroxolyn) is especially useful in this situation. Thiazides increase calcium reabsorption, which is the opposite effect that loop diuretics have on calcium. Because the reabsorption of calcium allows less calcium to enter the urinary tract, the thiazides have the additional indication for nephrolithiasis due to hypercalciuria. Thiazides are also used to alleviate the hypernatremia that is associated with nephrogenic diabetes insipidus.

Potassium-sparing diuretics are less efficacious in treating hypertension, but are useful in preventing hypokalemia induced by loop or thiazide diuretics. They are also indicated in severe heart failure and in post-MI patients with CHF symptoms and an EF of less than 40% to reduce mortality. Noncardiac uses include hyperaldosteronism.

Contraindications and Precautions

Patients who are allergic to sulfonamides may have cross reactivity with loop and thiazide diuretics.

Potassium-sparing agents may cause life-threatening hyperkalemia, so potassium supplementation should not be used concomitantly. Avoid use in renal impairment, which contributes to potassium retention. Exercise extreme caution with other medications that block the renin-angiotensin-aldosterone system. Dosage should be adjusted in hepatic impairment.

Adverse Reactions

- The thiazide and loop diuretics have the following effects on electrolytes: hypokalemia, hyponatremia, and hypomagnesemia.
- The potassium-sparing diuretics retain potassium (as their name implies); their potential effect on electrolytes is hyperkalemia and hyponatremia.
- Myalgias and muscle fatigue may result from hypokalemia and hypomagnesemia, which may occur with the thiazide or loop diuretics.
- Potentially deadly cardiac arrhythmias may occur in severe hypokalemia and hypomagnesemia.
- Insulin resistance worsens with thiazide diuretics.
- Hypertriglyceridemia and hypercholesterolemia may also occur, but are less prominent with loop diuretics.
- Hyperuricemia may occur; this may precipitate gout or nephrolithiasis.
- Loop diuretics may cause hypocalcemia, which the other agents do not cause.
- Loop diuretics may also cause ototoxicity.
- Weakness, fatigue, and paresthesias may also occur with diuretic use.

Drug Interactions

Lithium levels may increase with concomitant diuretic use, leading to possible toxicity.

NSAIDs reduce prostaglandin synthesis. Because loop, thiazide, and potassium-sparing diuretics rely on the action of prostaglandin within the kidney, NSAIDs reduce the effectiveness of these diuretics.

Drugs that inhibit the hepatic metabolizing system, cytochrome P450 3A4 isoenzyme, significantly increase levels of eplerenone.

Miscellaneous

Diuretics work synergistically with other agents to lower blood pressure. Many antihypertensive agents cause a compensatory increase in sodium and fluid retention, which is countered by the addition of a diuretic.

Limiting the dose of HCTZ or chlorthalidone to 12.5–25 mg daily significantly reduces the possibility of most of the metabolic side effects associated with diuretic usage.

Blood pressure, renal function (BUN and serum creatinine), and electrolytes (potassium, sodium, and magnesium) should be monitored at baseline, several weeks after initiation or titration of dosage, and routinely (once every 6–12 months) in patients on diuretic therapy. Additionally, uric acid levels should be monitored routinely in patients on thiazide diuretics.

Chapter 9

Digoxin

Mechanism of Action

Digoxin, a positive inotrope, is a cardiac glycoside that has several effects on the heart. It acts on the sodium pump to increase the intracellular concentration of calcium, which is then used to activate the contractile elements in the heart, thereby increasing contractility.

Although one would not expect a positive inotrope to combat the sympathetic nervous system, digoxin differs from other inotropes and does just that. Digoxin reduces the excessive sympathetic stimulation that is partially to blame for the progression of heart failure and for increased mortality in heart-failure patients.

Because digoxin reduces sympathetic stimulation and increases parasympathetic activity, it reduces heart rate. This helps increase diastolic filling time to augment preload. It also prolongs AV nodal refractoriness, thereby slowing conduction through the AV node.

Indications

Because digoxin is both a positive inotrope and a negative chronotrope it is useful in both heart failure and in slowing the ventricular response in patients with atrial fibrillation.

Contraindications and Precautions

Digoxin has a narrow therapeutic window; if this threshold is exceeded, patients may develop toxicity. Electrolyte imbalances that result from diuretic use and renal insufficiency may predispose patients to the development of toxicity.

Exercise caution in patients with sinus bradycardia or AV block, PVCs, acute MI, chronic constrictive pericarditis, hypertrophic obstructive cardiomyopathy, renal insufficiency, severe pulmonary disease, or hypothyroidism.

Adverse Reactions

Digoxin is generally well tolerated, but can cause a wide variety of adverse effects, which include the following:

- GI complaints such as anorexia, diarrhea, nausea, and vomiting
- CNS complaints such as fatigue, headache, confusion, and visual disturbances
- Visual disturbances such as seeing halos, having difficulty with color perception, or photophobia
- Any type of arrhythmia
- Hallucinations or delirium

> **Pearl**
> Arrhythmias are potentially life threatening and may be the first manifestation of toxicity so take great care to know the drug interactions in an effort to prevent toxicity. Electrolyte disturbances and impaired renal function predispose patients to toxicity so be sure to monitor for these conditions as well.

Drug Interactions

Digoxin has many drug interactions and toxicity may occur, so close attention to interactions and dosing is essential.

Antiarrhythmic drugs such as amiodarone and quinidine and the CCBs verapamil, nifedipine, and diltiazem may increase digoxin levels leading to toxicity. Cut the dose of digoxin in half and check a digoxin level several days after adding one of these antiarrhythmic agents to the regimen.

Substances that alter electrolytes may predispose patients to digoxin toxicity. These substances include diuretics, glucagon, amphotericin B, carbenicillin and ticarcillin, corticosteroids, laxatives, dextrose-insulin infusions, and large doses of dextrose.

Drug interactions that interfere with the renal excretion of digoxin may lead to toxicity.

Antibiotics alter the normal gut flora. Digoxin is partially metabolized by gut flora, so a course of antibiotics may result in a significant elevation of the digoxin level. Check a digoxin level after adding a macrolide antibiotic or an antifungal to the patient's regimen.

IV calcium, succinylcholine, and sympathomimetics, which are found in many OTC cold preparations as well as ephedrine, epinephrine, and isoproterenol may precipitate arrhythmias.

Antacids, bile acid sequestrants, cytotoxic drugs, and radiation may impair the absorption of digoxin.

Miscellaneous

Lanoxicaps are better absorbed than digoxin, so lower doses are used.

When ordering a digoxin level, wait 6 hours after the last dose was taken, otherwise levels will appear falsely elevated. It is easiest to achieve this by having the level drawn first thing in the morning before the medication is given.

Digoxin immune Fab (Digibind) is administered for life-threatening digoxin toxicity in addition to other measures.

Check heart rate, rhythm, blood pressure, and electrolytes prior to initiation. Monitor renal function, heart rhythm, and electrolytes closely while on digoxin.

Therapeutic levels range from 0.5 to 2.0 ng/ml. Patients with heart failure are typically maintained at a level less than 1.0 ng/ml.

Patients should not take an extra dose of digoxin if they miss a dose.

If nausea, vomiting, or diarrhea occur, the patient is more prone to toxicity and a digoxin level and electrolyte panel may be indicated.

Chapter 10

Antiplatelet Agents

Aspirin

Mechanism of Action

Thromboxane A2 is a prostaglandin that causes platelet aggregation; aspirin acts on the enzyme cyclooxygenase to inhibit the synthesis of thromboxane A2. The effect of aspirin on the platelets is irreversible, so the effect remains for the life of the platelet (about 8 to 10 days). Other nonsteroidal anti-inflammatory medications (NSAIDs) also inhibit the enzyme cyclooxygenase, but their effects are reversible.

Indications

Despite the availability of more expensive antiplatelet agents, aspirin is still the preferred agent in the treatment of acute coronary syndrome. Aspirin also reduces the rate of recurrent MI, stroke, and death in the post-MI patient. This is why all patients, unless contraindicated, should be discharged on aspirin after sustaining an MI and remain on it indefinitely.

Contraindications and Precautions

Aspirin is contraindicated in patients with G6PD deficiency, bleeding disorders, and if hypersensitivity to aspirin or NSAIDs has occurred in the past. Exercise caution in patients with impaired hepatic or renal function, thrombotic thrombocytopenic purpura, vitamin K deficiency, GI lesions, or hypoprothrombinemia.

Aspirin should never be given to children with chickenpox or flu-like symptoms because of the potential to cause Reye's syndrome.

Adverse Reactions

- Anaphylaxis
- Dyspepsia/GI bleeding
- Thrombocytopenia
- Ototoxicity

Drug Interactions

Other antiplatelet, anticoagulant, or thrombolytic agents may increase the risk of bleeding if used concomitantly.

Aspirin interferes with the renal clearance of lithium, thereby raising lithium levels leading to potential toxicity.

Antibiotics, corticosteroids, and other GI irritants may increase the potential for adverse GI effects.

Miscellaneous

Educate the patient about the increased risk of bleeding and signs and symptoms that may indicate a GI bleed (i.e. melena).

Discontinue aspirin 1 week prior to surgery if bleeding is a concern.

Chronic aspirin therapy results in about a 2% risk of major bleeding. However, lower doses (75 to 162 mg) have lower rates of bleeding and are now recommended.

Monitor the platelet count with a baseline CBC and repeat this every 6 months.

Clopidogrel

Mechanism of Action

Clopidogrel (Plavix) and ticlodipine (Ticlid) both irreversibly inhibit a receptor on platelets, thereby inhibiting platelet aggregation. Neither of these drugs affects the prostaglandins. Ticlodipine is rarely used in clinical practice.

Indications

Clopidogrel is recommended in acute coronary syndrome or for secondary prevention post-MI in those who are allergic to aspirin. It is also administered after cardiac stenting to reduce the risk of restenosis.

Contraindications and Precautions

Clopidogrel is contraindicated in patients with intracranial hemorrhage, peptic ulcer disease, or other conditions with active bleeding. Exercise caution in patients with recent trauma or surgery because they are at risk for bleeding. Caution is also necessary in patients with hepatic impairment.

Adverse Reactions

- Ticlopidine causes leukopenia in 1% of recipients and therefore requires monitoring of the blood count regularly. For this reason, clopidogrel has essentially replaced it in clinical practice.
- Clopidogrel is generally well tolerated. GI symptoms, rash or pruritis, and purpura may occur.
- CNS complaints such as dizziness, fatigue, or paresthesias may also result.

Interactions

Other antiplatelet or anticoagulant agents may increase the risk of bleeding.

Miscellaneous

Educate the patient about the increased risk of bleeding and signs and symptoms that may indicate a GI bleed (i.e. melena).

If the patient develops toxicity as indicated by a GI bleed, vomiting, or difficulty breathing, consider platelet transfusion if clinically indicated.

Monitor the platelet count with a baseline CBC and repeat this every 6 months.

Chapter 11

Antiarrhythmics

There are four classes of antiarrhythmic drugs based on the primary effect the agent has on the action potential (Vaughan Williams Classification). The action potential is the electrical activity that occurs in the cells of muscles or nerves in response to mechanical, chemical, or electrical stimulation. Channels in the cardiac cell membrane open and close at different times during the action potential allowing ions (Na^+, K^+, Ca^{++}) to pass through the cell membrane and create an electrical current.

Mechanism of Action

Type I agents block sodium channels. Type II agents, beta-blockers, inhibit the sympathetic nervous system. Type III agents prolong the duration of the action potential; the type III agents, sotalol (Betapace) and dofetilide (Tikosyn), accomplish this by prolonging the QT interval. Type IV agents, calcium channel blockers, block the entry of calcium into the cell, thereby slowing conduction, decreasing automaticity of the SA and AV node, and prolonging refractoriness.

Some medications may exert more than one of these effects or have metabolites that exert a different class of action. For instance, sotalol is a nonselective beta-blocker categorized as a type III antiarrhythmic because of its effect on the action potential.

Indications

Type Ia drugs are effective in both supraventricular and ventricular arrhythmias, but toxicity has virtually eliminated their use in clinical practice. Type Ib drugs are significantly more effective in ventricular arrhythmias than supraventricular arrhythmias. Type Ic agents are effective in preventing episodes of PSVT or atrial fibrillation, but their use in ventricular arrhythmias has been limited by the potential for proarrhythmias.

Type II and IV agents are both effective in slowing the ventricular rate in atrial tachycardias and in treating automatic or reentrant tachycardias that arise from the SA or AV node. Esmolol, a parenteral type II agent, is often used after surgery to control ventricular rate in atrial fibrillation and atrial flutter.

The type III agents, amiodarone and sotalol, are effective in most tachycardias. Amiodarone is indicated for prevention and treatment of ventricular fibrillation and recurrent unstable ventricular tachycardia. It is also the drug of choice in cardiac arrest. Although not FDA approved for atrial fibrillation, amiodarone is effective in preventing recurrences of atrial fibrillation and can convert atrial fibrillation to sinus rhythm. Sotalol is used for atrial fibrillation as well as for ventricular arrhythmias. Bretylium, another type III agent, is often used in VF but not VT because it increases the VF threshold but does not have antitachycardia effects.

Adenosine is an antiarrhythmic that is not classified by the Vaughan Williams Classification scheme. It is highly effective in converting supraventricular arrhythmias and is preferred over CCBs for this purpose. It is not useful in atrial fibrillation, atrial flutter, or multifocal tachycardia.

Selecting an Antiarrhythmic

Quinidine, procainamide (Pronestyl), and disopyramide (Norpace) are examples of type Ia antiarrhythmics. Lidocaine, mexiletine, and tocainide are type Ib agents, which are administered by IV because of their short half-lives. Flecainide (Tambocor) and propafenone (Rythmol) are type Ic agents.

The beta-blockers propranolol (Inderal), acebutolol (Sectral), and esmolol (Brevibloc) are indicated for the treatment of arrhythmias.

Type III agents include sotalol (Betapace), dofetilide (Tikosyn), amiodarone (Cordarone, Pacerone), bretylium, and ibutilide.

Type IV agents, CCBs, are discussed in Chapter 5.

Contraindications and Precautions

All antiarrhythmics are also proarrhythmic. Patients with underlying heart disease such as coronary artery disease or congestive heart failure are at increased risk of proarrhythmia and have increased mortality rates with type Ic agents. Therefore, these agents are reserved for patients with no evidence of heart disease.

Type Ic agents can cause slow atrial flutter with the possibility of a rapid ventricular response. To prevent this possibility, an AV-nodal blocker (beta-blocker, nondihydropyridine CCB, or digoxin) must be administered concomitantly.

Patients who are in atrial fibrillation or flutter that have Wolff-Parkinson-White syndrome should not be given any AV-nodal blocking agents such as CCBs, digoxin, or adenosine. If the AV-nodal conduction is blocked by one of these agents, conduction may proceed down the accessory pathway instead. This may result in extremely rapid ventricular rates.

> **Pearl**
>
> To ensure the selection of the safest and least toxic antiarrhythmic agent, perform an echocardiogram and an ischemic evaluation to assess for underlying ischemia or structural heart disease prior to selecting an antiarrhythmic medication.

Adverse Reactions

One of the most concerning adverse events associated with the administration of antiarrhythmics is the development of torsades de pointes. The risk of developing this malignant dysrhythmia while taking a QT-prolonging medication is increased in the setting of hypokalemia, hypomagnesemia, bradycardia, and with higher doses of the medication.

Type Ia drugs have fallen out of favor due to excess toxicity because they all may cause torsades de pointes due to QT prolongation. Procainamide causes a lupus-like syndrome in up to 30% of patients. Disopyramide causes significant and bothersome anticholinergic side effects and may worsen heart failure.

Patients on amiodarone must be closely monitored for adverse reactions such as pulmonary fibrosis, thyroid dysfunction, hepatic necrosis, and optic neuritis. Therefore, you should obtain baseline thyroid function tests, liver function tests, and a chest X-ray and repeat these studies every 3 to 6 months. Additionally, you should ensure that the patient undergoes an annual eye exam. These severe reactions may be irreversible and can be fatal. They can occur at the 200 mg daily dose commonly used for atrial fibrillation, but are more common with higher doses such as the 400 mg daily dose used for ventricular arrhythmias.

Amiodarone may also cause GI upset, skin reactions such as a blue-gray discoloration, bradyarrhythmias, and peripheral neuropathy. Because of toxicity issues, other antiarrhythmics are commonly employed first-line. Amiodarone is typically reserved for patients with underlying structural heart disease or congestive heart failure who are prone to higher mortality rates with the use of other antiarrhythmics. Although amiodarone prolongs the QT interval, torsades de pointes is uncommon and therefore patients are often placed on amiodarone in an outpatient setting.

> **Pearl**
>
> The treatment of torsades de pointes is magnesium sulfate 1–2 grams IV over 5–60 minutes.

Drug Interactions

When instituting amiodarone, it is important to reduce the dose of digoxin and check a digoxin level soon afterward. This is because amiodarone can increase serum concentrations of digoxin leading to potential toxicity.

Amiodarone also potentiates the effect of beta-blockers, some CCBs, warfarin, and other antiarrythmics.

Dofetilide has many drug interactions and must be administered with caution.

> **Pearl**
>
> If you encounter a patient with SVT, give a trial of carotid sinus massage after carefully assessing the patient to ensure they have no carotid bruits. This maneuver may be therapeutic in the setting of SVT and is also diagnostic in the setting of atrial flutter, by slowing the ventricular response so that you can identify the flutter waves.

SECTION II RESOURCES

Abramowicz, Mark, et al. 2004. "Drugs for Cardiac Arrhythmias." *The Medical Letter*. 2(27):75–82.

Abramowicz, Mark, et al. 2005. "Drugs for Hypertension." *The Medical Letter*. 3(34):39–48.

Abramowicz, Mark, et al. 2001. "Which Beta-Blocker?" *The Medical Letter*. 43(1097):9–11.

DiPiro, Joseph T., Robert L. Talbert, Gary C. Yee, et al. 2005. *Pharmacotherapy: A Pathophysiologic Approach*. 6th ed. New York, NY: McGraw Hill.

Furberg, Carl D., and Bruce M Psaty. *Should Evidence-Based Proof of Drug Efficacy Be Extrapolated to a "Class of Agents"?* Retrieved from http://circ.ahajournals.org/cgi/content/full/108/21/2608. Accessed January 6, 2007.

Katzung, Bertram G. 2004. *Basic and Clinical Pharmacology*. 9th ed. New York, NY: McGraw-Hill Companies.

Kendall, Martin. 1997. "Clinical Relevance of Pharmacokinetic Differences Between Beta Blockers." *The American Journal of Cardiology*. 80(9B):155–195.

Physician's Drug Handbook. 9th ed. 2001. Philadelphia, PA: Springhouse

Cardio Consults

Physician assistants (PAs) and nurse practitioners (NPs) are often asked to see patients who present with symptoms that may reflect underlying cardiac disorders. When seeing the patient in consultation, first determine the reason you have been asked to see the patient. This sounds straightforward, but often the patient's most urgent or apparent problem is not the real reason for the consultation. For example, a patient who clearly needs evaluation of ischemic symptoms may be sent for preoperative clearance. Always be aware of the reason you have been asked to see the patient.

When dealing with a potential cardiac disorder, promptly assess how critical the patient is before performing a comprehensive evaluation. Active, acute, or progressively worsening symptoms may indicate the need for acute intervention. Unstable vital signs, acute mental status changes, and acute EKG changes may also indicate critical cardiac disease.

If you are in an outpatient setting and determine that the patient is critical, you may need to call the EMS to transport the patient to the hospital. If in an inpatient setting, it may be necessary to transfer the patient to the ICU and consult the critical care team. If the patient is not in acute distress, you can begin the standard evaluation utilizing history, the physical exam, and basic studies. Chest pain, shortness of breath, palpitations, dizziness, syncope, and edema are symptoms that are often addressed in clinical practice and are discussed in this section.

Chapter 12

Chest Pain

Introduction

The most common causes of chest pain (CP) in patients who present to primary care providers are musculoskeletal conditions, GI disorders, stable coronary heart disease (CHD), panic disorder, and pulmonary conditions. Although life-threatening cardiac conditions rarely present to primary care providers, one must be vigilant to exclude these disorders.

The picture changes when patients present to the emergency department (ED). More than 50% of patients who present to the ED with CP have a diagnosis of MI, angina, heart failure, or pulmonary embolism (PE).

Although there are many benign etiologies of CP, potentially life-threatening causes should be ruled out. These include acute coronary syndrome, aortic dissection, and pulmonary embolism. With so many patients admitted for "CP: Rule out MI," it is important to maintain a high index of suspicion so as not to overlook the rare PE or aortic dissection.

Differential Diagnosis

Common cardiac causes of CP include myocardial ischemia or infarction, aortic dissection, valvular heart disease, pericarditis, and myocarditis.

Aortic dissection is a life-threatening condition that requires a high index of suspicion. It is described as a sudden, severe, "ripping" or "tearing" sensation, which is not pleuritic or positional. Pain is typically located in the center of the chest (with ascending dissection) or in the back (with descending dissection). It is most common in men older than age 60; hypertension is the most important risk factor. The EKG will typically appear normal, but a chest X-ray may reveal a widened mediastinum. A CT scan, MRI, TEE, or aortography can confirm the diagnosis.

Aortic stenosis has a classic triad of CP, dyspnea, and syncope. Patients may present with any of, or a combination of, these symptoms and will have a characteristic heart murmur. Listen carefully for this murmur in all patients presenting with CP because stress testing, which is often employed in the evaluation of CP, is contraindicated in patients with significant aortic stenosis.

The CP of pericarditis is pleuritic, which is sharp and worsens with inspiration or movement, and patients feel better when leaning forward. A pericardial friction rub may be audible and the patient may be febrile. The EKG will reveal widespread ST segment elevation with no reciprocal changes.

Myocarditis is an inflammatory disorder that may result from infectious, toxic, or autoimmune insults. It may be accompanied by heart failure symptoms such as dyspnea and/or systemic symptoms such as fever and myalgias. CP may also accompany this disorder and may be difficult to differentiate from ischemic pain.

The presentation of myocardial ischemia will be reviewed later. Acute coronary syndrome will be discussed in detail in Chapter 19.

Because the heart and esophagus share similar neurologic innervation, the pain of these organ systems is often indistinguishable. For this reason, any patient with cardiac risk factors who presents with typical features of ischemic CP should have myocardial ischemia ruled out before chest pain is attributed to a GI cause.

Gastroesophageal reflux disease may cause CP that is characteristic of angina, but patients usually have additional complaints of dyspepsia, regurgitation, acid taste, or burning. Also, GI-related chest pain may be related to meals. Although a trial of acid suppression may assist in making the diagnosis, always perform a cardiac evaluation as well.

Pulmonary causes of CP, of which there are many, typically present with pleuritic pain. A chest X-ray will help to exclude many of these causes of chest pain such as a pneumothorax or pneumonia.

An important pulmonary disorder to consider in your differential diagnosis is pulmonary embolus (PE) because it is a potentially life-threatening condition. It should be considered in any patient who presents with chest pain or dyspnea that is not fully explained by the initial evaluation including a thorough H&P, Chest X-ray, and EKG. A PE is more likely if one or more of the following risk factors are present: immobilization, surgery within the last 3 months, recent stroke, or a history of venous thromboembolism or malignancy. You may hear a loud pulmonic component (P2) of the second heart sound if the acute increase in pulmonary vascular resistance leads to right-sided heart failure. However, the physical exam will often offer no clues. Musculoskeletal abnormalities may cause chest pain as well. Movement, position changes, or palpation often provoke these disorders. The most common musculoskeletal cause of chest pain is costochondritis. This condition is usually identified by reproduction of chest pain when palpating along the costochondral joints of the chest wall during the physical exam.

CP may also be attributed to emotional or psychiatric conditions. This pain is usually nonexertional and may persist more than 30 minutes or may be accompanied by other signs of an emotional disorder. It is important to identify cardiac risk factors in these patients and exclude underlying ischemia if warranted. A psychiatric etiology is a diagnosis of exclusion in the CP patient.

The most important tool to guide your decision making and aid in the proper use of diagnostic studies is a well-conducted history and physical.

Historical Questions to Narrow Your Differential

Does the Patient Have a History of Cardiac Disease or Other Vascular Disease?

If the patient has a history of angina, ask them if their current symptoms are the same as, or different from, their prior angina pain.

A stenosis in one artery makes other arteries likely to be affected. Therefore, always perform a thorough investigation, in both your H&P exam, for cerebrovascular disease (one-sided weakness, diplopia, slurred speech), carotid artery disease (decreased carotid upstroke, carotid bruits), and peripheral vascular disease (symptoms of intermittent claudication, poor pedal pulses). Don't forget that diabetes mellitus is a cardiovascular risk equivalent because these patients are practically guaranteed to have concomitant vascular disease.

Where Is the Discomfort Located and Does It Radiate?

Angina, the term used to describe the classic presentation of ischemic chest pain, is typically a diffuse discomfort that may be difficult to localize. The patient often indicates a large area of the chest, rather than a localized area, when asked where the discomfort is felt. Radiation to the neck, jaw, and shoulder are common.

> **Pearl**
>
> Patients often struggle to describe the location and quality of their discomfort and instead place their fists over their chests in an effort to describe it. This is known as the Levine sign and is a classic presentation of ischemic pain.

When Did the Discomfort Begin, How Often Does It Occur, and How Long Does Each Episode Last?

Angina generally lasts for 2 to 5 minutes. It is not a fleeting discomfort that lasts only for a few seconds or less than a minute. On the other hand, it generally will not last for 20 to 30 minutes or longer unless the patient is experiencing an acute myocardial infarction.

Angina occurs more commonly in the early morning due to an increase in sympathetic tone, which increases myocardial oxygen demand.

> **Pearl**
>
> Patients often describe their pain as sharp because it is severe, not because the quality is sharp. Be sure you understand what the patient means by this adjective.

What Does the Discomfort Feel Like?

Ischemic chest pain is generally not sharp, but rather dull or aching.

Phrases patients will often use to describe ischemic pain include:

- Squeezing
- Tightness
- Pressure
- Constriction
- Strangling
- Burning or heartburn
- Fullness in the chest
- Band-like sensation around chest; for women, as if their "bras are too tight"
- Knot in the center of the chest
- Lump in throat
- Ache
- Heavy weight on chest (elephant sitting on chest)
- Toothache

> **Pearl**
>
> Patients may vehemently deny having chest pain; some even get upset if you continue to call their "discomfort" chest pain. I always ask, "Do you have any pressure, pain, or discomfort in your chest?"

On a Scale of 1 to 10, 10 Being Most Severe, How Would You Rate Your Pain?

This scale will help to assess response to treatment and should be recorded after each intervention.

What Are the Associated Symptoms?

The most common symptoms associated with ischemic chest pain are shortness of breath, belching, nausea/vomiting, diaphoresis or clamminess, dizziness or lightheadedness, and fatigue.

Cardio Reality

I arrive at the ED in response to an urgent page; the ED physician explains that the patient presented with chest pain, ST elevation in the anterior leads of his EKG, and elevation of his initial cardiac enzymes.

The ED physician hands me the chart and I quickly review the EKG, CXR report, and lab results while calling the catheterization lab to notify them that the patient needs to be taken to the lab urgently as he is having an anterior MI.

I hang up the phone and enter the patient's room to perform a directed history and physical in a matter of minutes. As I finish up my rapid assessment, the catheterization team arrives as if on cue. I begin to explain the urgency of the patient's condition to the patient and his family.

The patient interrupts me with a puzzled look on his face, "What are you talking about? I am just having indigestion!" I smile as I think to myself, "here we go again." Many patients believe they are having indigestion when they are actually suffering from an MI. It is very difficult to distinguish between the two. For this reason, it is prudent to always consider a cardiac etiology in patients who present with "indigestion."

In What Setting Does the Chest Pain Occur? Does Anything Provoke or Exacerbate It?

Activities and situations that increase myocardial oxygen demand will provoke or exacerbate ischemia. Chest pain brought on by exertion or stress is the classic presentation of angina. Ischemic chest pain does not change with respiration or position.

> **Bottom Line**
>
> Typical angina pain is described as substernal, provoked by exertion, and relieved by rest or nitroglycerine.

What Relieves the Pain?

Factors that reduce oxygen demand or increase oxygen supply will result in relief of angina. These include cessation of activity, use of nitrates, sitting upright, Valsalva maneuver, and/or carotid sinus pressure. Keep in mind that nitrates also relieve the discomfort associated with esophageal spasm.

Inquire About Cardiac Risk Factors

Ask whether the patient has a history of hypertension, dyslipidemia, tobacco use, diabetes mellitus, or a sedentary lifestyle. Also inquire whether the patient has a family history of premature ischemic heart disease.

Bottom Line

Historical findings that decrease the likelihood of an ischemic etiology include chest pain that is pleuritic, localized with one finger, reproduced by palpation or movement, lasts less than a few seconds, or radiates to the lower extremities or above the mandible.

Physical Exam

Although the physical exam may be entirely normal, some clues that the chest pain may have a cardiac etiology include an increase in the heart rate, an elevation in blood pressure, new heart sounds, new murmurs or changes in preexisting murmurs, or abnormal precordial movements.

General: When conducting your physical exam, remember to first ensure that the patient is not in shock or acute distress. Look for cyanosis, pallor, or diaphoresis.

HEENT: Inspect the eyes for xanthelasma (yellow plaques near the inner eyelid, which may be associated with elevated lipid levels) or arcus senilis (an opaque, cloudy arc or circle around the edge of the iris, which may signify an increased risk of coronary artery disease when present in younger people).

Lungs: Pulmonary auscultation may identify congestive heart failure, asthma, COPD, or pneumonia.

Cardiac: Inspect (you may see evidence of herpes zoster) and palpate (you may reproduce the pain of costochondritis) the chest wall for any evidence of musculoskeletal causes of CP. Also palpate the PMI and for any heaves or thrills. Auscultate for any abnormal heart sounds or murmurs.

Abdomen: The abdominal exam may suggest peptic ulcer disease (PUD), cholecystitis, or pancreatitis.

Diagnostic Strategy and Management

The EKG is an important tool in the evaluation of chest pain, but remember that the EKG may appear entirely normal in patients who are experiencing ischemic pain, especially if the patient is not having active symptoms at the time of the study. Ischemia and infarcts are usually, but not always, identified by ST- t wave abnormalities on the EKG. A new onset bundle branch block (BBB) may also indicate an MI. Pericarditis is associated with diffuse ST elevation. Arrhythmias are often identified on the EKG as well.

The chest radiograph is an integral part of the chest pain evaluation. Consider ordering a chest X-ray on all patients with "Chest Pain: Rule out MI" to be sure there is no widened mediastinum of aortic dissection. When the initial presentation gives you a higher index of suspicion for aortic dissection, consider ordering a chest CT instead. The chest X-ray also helps to identify pulmonary edema, cardiomegaly, pleural effusions, and pericardial effusions.

Beneficial lab studies include a CBC to detect anemia, which may exacerbate ischemia. A chemistry panel is useful for assessment of renal function, electrolytes, and hydration status. If you are concerned about hypoxia, consider an ABG. If you are concerned about a GI cause, check liver function tests and a serum amylase and lipase.

Cardiac enzymes (CK, CK-MB, and troponin) should be ordered stat and serially (every 6 to 8 hours) within a 24-hour period to determine if an infarction has occurred. If the patient presents with symptoms that began very recently, you may also want to order a myoglobin level which may become elevated as soon as 1 hour after an infarction. It can take up to 3 hours for the CK-MB or troponin level to rise after an infarct and the CK-MB levels don't peak until 8–10 hours after the event. Troponin levels have a biphasic pattern of release and take even longer to reach their peak levels, first at about 14 hours and again at 3 to 5 days after the infarction has occurred.

> **Pearl**
>
> If you have a high enough index of suspicion to order cardiac enzymes, then you must order them over a 24-hour period. Never order just one set!

An echocardiogram will detect wall motion abnormalities in patients too acutely ill to undergo stress testing or catheterization. An echocardiogram will also detect valvular heart disease, pericardial effusions as in pericarditis, and ventricular dysfunction.

A stat CT or MRI may be indicated to exclude aortic dissection if clinically suspected.

If clinically indicated, a D-dimer level, ventilation-perfusion scan (V/Q scan), or a spiral CT may be needed to assess for pulmonary embolus.

If the patient has ruled out for MI by serial cardiac enzymes and EKGs, but ischemia is suggested by the initial evaluation, stress testing with or without imaging may be performed. This is usually performed prior to discharge.

Cardiac catheterization should be performed urgently in patients who rule in for an MI. It is also useful to assess patients with significant cardiac risk factors who present with classic angina symptoms and EKG abnormalities.

If cardiac catheterization and percutaneous transluminal coronary angioplasty (PTCA) are not readily available and the patient is having an acute ST elevation infarction, thrombolysis should be considered as discussed in Chapter 20.

Chapter 13

Dyspnea

Introduction

Dyspnea is a subjective complaint that is described differently by each patient. It may be described as shortness of breath, difficulty getting a deep breath, or a sensation of suffocation. Some people even describe it as a tightness, which may confuse this symptom with chest pain. Its formal interpretation is that of an uncomfortable awareness of one's breathing.

Differential Diagnosis

Cardiac conditions that may cause dyspnea include ischemia, congestive heart failure, pericardial effusion, valvular heart disease, or arrhythmias. Noncardiac causes of shortness of breath must be considered as well. Dyspnea may be caused by a pulmonary disorder such as asthma, COPD, pulmonary hypertension, pulmonary embolus, pneumonia, bronchitis, pneumothorax, anaphylaxis, aspiration, or interstitial lung disease. Other causes include anxiety or panic disorder, anemia, or acidosis.

Historical Questions to Narrow Your Differential

Was the Onset Sudden or Gradual?

Sudden onset may be caused by acute pulmonary edema, pneumothorax, pulmonary embolism, or airway obstruction. An acute episode of congestive heart failure or angina may also cause sudden onset of dyspnea; these conditions are frequently precipitated by exertion.

Gradual onset is seen more commonly in patients with COPD, chronic CHF, pneumonia, pleural effusion, pregnancy, or obesity. Asthma or obstructive airway disease is often accompanied by wheezing and the patient may report a history of improvement with bronchodilators.

What Are the Associated Symptoms?

Paroxysmal nocturnal dyspnea (PND) is episodic shortness of breath that occurs 2 to 4 hours after going to sleep and improves after sitting upright in bed. It is associated with diaphoresis, cough, and sometimes wheezing. It represents interstitial pulmonary edema, which is most commonly due to CHF.

Orthopnea is shortness of breath while recumbent. Patients are more comfortable sleeping in a recliner or propped up on pillows. Ask the patient how many pillows it takes to breathe comfortably. This is due to pulmonary venous congestion and is commonly a symptom of heart failure.

Angina, MI, PE, pneumonia, and pneumothorax may have concomitant chest pain. Pneumonia, asthma, or COPD may have associated coughing or wheezing. If the patient has associated anxiety, then anxiety disorder may be the culprit. CHF patients often have dependent edema or nocturia. Cough is commonly associated with pulmonary causes of dyspnea, but do not forget that a dry cough is a common adverse reaction of ACE inhibitors.

What Are the Precipitating or Relieving Factors?

Dyspnea precipitated by exertion may be related to ischemia or CHF.

What If the Patient's Significant Other Complains that the Patient Stops Breathing at Night?

Sleep apnea, which is common in overweight patients, is described as episodes of snoring with periods of apnea. Because sleep apnea can lead to pulmonary hypertension and is common in cardiac patients, screen all patients for this condition.

Cheyne-Stokes respiration is common in elderly patients with heart failure and is described as hyperpnea, an abnormal increase in rate and depth of breathing, followed by apnea, a brief cessation or marked reduction of breathing.

Physical Exam

When a thorough physical exam is impractical, the following elements of a cursory exam should suffice:

Vital signs: Include weight and oxygen saturation with vital signs.

General: Look for any evidence of respiratory distress. This includes respiratory rate, retraction, excessive use of accessory muscles of respiration, and cyanosis.

Skin: Assess skin color for cyanosis or pallor and look for diaphoresis.

Neck: Check for JVD, which is a sign of heart failure.

Lungs: Auscultate the lungs for adventitious sounds such as wheezes, rhonchi, or rales.

Heart: Perform a complete cardiac exam including auscultation for heart murmurs or extra heart sounds.

Extremities: Assess for clubbing, cyanosis, or edema.

Pearl

Documenting the patient's general appearance and whether or not they are in any respiratory distress is very important for your protection in the event of a poor outcome that may result in legal proceedings.

Diagnostic Strategy and Management

Provide supplemental oxygen or consult the respiratory/pulmonary service if mechanical ventilation is indicated. Order a CXR, EKG, CBC, chemistry panel, and a BNP (if you are unable to differentiate between CHF and pulmonary disease). Also, consider an ABG if you are worried about hypoxia. Rule out pulmonary embolus with a D-dimer, spiral CT, or V-Q scan.

Pearl

Always maintain a high index of suspicion for a PE!

Order stat and serial cardiac enzymes (troponin, CK, CK-MB) if you suspect that dyspnea is due to an MI. Remember that dyspnea may be the only sign of ischemia or infarct, especially in women or patients with diabetes mellitus.

An echocardiogram will provide an estimate of the ejection fraction if left ventricular dysfunction is a consideration. It will also identify the presence of valvular heart disease or wall motion abnormalities that may result from an infarction.

Consider pulmonary function testing if you are concerned about the possibility of chronic obstructive pulmonary disease.

Cardio Reality

I saw a 39-year-old woman for a follow-up of a CHF exacerbation. Upon reviewing her chart, I observed that she had suffered a massive anterior MI 2 years ago at the age of 37. I have seen several young women with cardiomyopathy, usually postpartum or viral, but never as a result of an MI. I was bothered by the fact that such a young woman had sustained such a devastating blow to her left ventricular function and thus her quality of life and prognosis.

During her visit, I inquired further about the circumstances surrounding her heart attack. It turns out that she had presented to several medical providers over the month preceding her MI with complaints of dyspnea on exertion. Because of her young age, the possibility of cardiac disease was never explored. She was told she had asthma and was treated with everything under the sun including prednisone. She finally got so sick she presented in florid pulmonary edema with an ejection fraction of less than 20% and evidence of a previous massive anterior MI. Now she is disabled and spends most of her time navigating between her medical appointments. It is heartbreaking to think that if her providers had included a cardiac evaluation of her dyspnea, this tragedy may have been avoided.

Chapter 14

Syncope

Introduction

Syncope is the transient loss of postural tone and consciousness that results from inadequate perfusion to the brain. A full recovery occurs quickly after a syncopal event. Dizziness, lightheadedness, and near-syncope have a similar differential diagnosis and workup, but are usually associated with less pathological conditions than true syncope.

Differential Diagnosis

The most common cause of syncope is vasovagal syncope, followed by cardiac causes. In roughly one third of cases, the underlying etiology remains unknown.

Common cardiovascular causes of syncope include aortic stenosis, arrhythmias, and hypertrophic obstructive cardiomyopathy (HOCM). Some less common cardiovascular causes include pulmonary embolus, pulmonary hypertension, dissecting aortic aneurysm, subclavian steal, atrial myxoma, and cardiac tamponade.

Arrhythmias are the most common cause of cardiac syncope. Sinus bradycardia (either due to medications, intrinsic sinus node dysfunction, or high vagal tone as in vasovagal syncope), high-grade AV block, sustained VT, or SVT are the more common syncope-inducing arrhythmias. Atrial fibrillation rarely causes syncope unless the ventricular rate is rapid.

Aortic stenosis and hypertrophic obstructive cardiomyopathy both cause obstruction of blood flow (as do the less common atrial myxomas, pulmonary emboli, pulmonic stenosis, and idiopathic pulmonary arterial hypertension) and therefore may result in syncope. Aortic stenosis may present with chest pain, dyspnea, and/or syncope, the symptoms are typically exertional, and a characteristic heart murmur will be noted on exam. Syncope in patients with HOCM may be precipitated by reduced preload as in hypovolemia, use of certain medications such as diuretics or nitrates, and postural changes.

Noncardiovascular etiologies are typically associated with a good prognosis. Common noncardiovascular conditions that cause syncope include vasovagal (neurocardiogenic) syncope, carotid sinus hypersensitivity, situational syncope, orthostatic hypotension, and psychogenic disorders. Some less-common noncardiac causes of syncope include hyperventilation or migraines. Syncope is often mistaken for conditions such as seizures, alcohol- or drug-induced loss of consciousness, strokes, or hypoglycemia.

> **Pearl**
>
> Ventricular fibrillation does not cause syncope; it causes cardiac arrest and/or sudden death.

Neurocardiogenic syncope is commonly seen in young people and has a prodrome of fatigue, nausea, diaphoresis, and pallor. Symptoms are typically precipitated by prolonged standing, heat exposure, exercise, or fear.

When pressure is exerted upon the carotid sinus, the vagus nerve can be stimulated. When the vagus nerve is stimulated, it causes activation of the parasympathetic nervous system (the opposite of the fight-or-flight response). This results in a decreased heart rate and decreased blood pressure. In carotid sinus hypersensitivity, minimal stimulus results in vagal stimulation and a dramatic reduction in blood pressure and pulse ensues, resulting in a syncopal spell. This is a relatively uncommon cause of syncope and is more commonly seen in older patients.

Situational syncope may be precipitated by coughing, defecation, blood drawing, postmicturition, or similar circumstances.

Orthostatic hypotension (a 20 mmHg or greater reduction in blood pressure when the patient goes from a recumbent position to an upright posture) may lead to syncope. It may be caused by volume depletion, autonomic dysfunction as seen in diabetes mellitus, or may be iatrogenic due to certain medications. Medications often implicated include tricyclic or phenothiazine antidepressants, opiates, bromocriptine, and antihypertensives.

Although the differential diagnosis is broad, several historical questions can narrow your focus.

Historical Questions to Narrow Your Differential

Because the patient becomes unconscious during a syncopal spell, it is helpful to direct some of these questions to any witnesses if present. Often times the witness will not be present but the patient will recall what the witness told them about the episode.

Was There an Aura or Warning Signs?

Sudden syncope with no warning is characteristic of cardiac syncope due to an arrhythmia. On the other hand, neurological causes typically are associated with premonitory nausea, diaphoresis, yawning, or abnormal vision or hearing. Patients who have a tachyarrhythmia may experience a rapid heartbeat or palpitations either associated with the episode or historically.

> **Pearl**
>
> Stokes-Adams syndrome is an example of abrupt loss of consciousness without warning. It is caused by complete heart block, sinus arrest, or ventricular tachyarrhythmias.

Did the Patient Have a Rapid Return to Normal Mentation or Were There Lingering Symptoms After the Syncopal Spell?

Postictal symptoms, such as confusion, are suggestive of seizure activity. Neurological deficits such as one-sided weakness, abnormal speech, or vision disorders are suggestive of cerebrovascular ischemia as in a CVA or TIA.

Was the Episode Associated with Bowel or Bladder Incontinence?

These symptoms are often associated with a seizure rather than a true syncopal spell.

Did the Patient Sustain Any Trauma to the Head or Neck?
Were Any Other Injuries Noted?

Syncopal spells due to arrhythmias often occur without any warning signs; therefore patients may sustain injuries during the attacks.

What Was the Patient Doing When the Episode Occurred?

Exertional syncope may be caused by a left ventricular outflow obstruction such as severe aortic stenosis or hypertrophic obstructive cardiomyopathy. Primary pulmonary hypertension may also present this way.

Syncope that occurs when patients rise from recumbency to an upright position suggests postural hypotension or vasovagal syncope. Postural hypotension may be secondary to volume depletion, medication side effects, autonomic dysfunction, or peripheral neuropathy.

In carotid sinus hypersensitivity, the patient reports wearing a tight collar or turning their head prior to the episode. Patients may report syncopal spells when they turn their head into the shoulder strap of their seatbelt.

Is There a Family History of Syncope or Sudden Death at a Young Age from Unknown or Cardiac Causes?

Congenital Long QT syndrome, right ventricular dysplasia, or HOCM may be the culprit if a family history of syncope is identified.

Physical Exam

A thorough physical exam is imperative in the evaluation of syncope.

Vital signs: Include orthostatic BP and pulse. Look for hypotension, tachycardia or bradycardia.

General: Be sure to look for any obvious injuries (lacerations, ecchmosis), neurological deficits (slurred speech, hemiparesis), or signs of shock (diaphoresis, pallor).

HEENT: Assess for abnormal carotid upstroke and/ or bruits that may signify cerebrovascular disease.

Lungs: Listen for rales that may signify an underlying cardiac cause.

Cardiac: A systolic ejection murmur may indicate AS or HOCM (having the patient squat or perform a Valsalva maneuver will help to differentiate between the two). A diastolic murmur may be present in aortic dissection or mitral stenosis. A loud P2 may indicate pulmonary embolus. A laterally displaced PMI may indicate underlying cardiomyopathy, which may predispose the patient to life-threatening arrhythmias.

Neurologic: Full assessment for any residual weakness or abnormalities is essential.

Diagnostic Strategy and Management

In many cases, the history, physical exam, and EKG will enable you to make a diagnosis of syncope and its cause. For instance, an elderly woman who has just had her ACE inhibitor titrated upward for better blood pressure control may present with frank syncopal spells preceded by dizziness and visual changes that occur when going from a seated position to standing. This history, accompanied by a reduction in blood pressure when standing on physical exam and a benign EKG, will enable you to comfortably make the diagnosis of orthostatic hypotension.

A firm diagnosis of syncope can be made in several situations. If syncope is precipitated by fear, severe pain, or emotional stress, prolonged standing, or with procedures such as blood drawing, a diagnosis of vasovagal syncope can be made with confidence. If syncope occurs during or immediately following urination, defecation, coughing, or swallowing, a diagnosis of situational syncope is appropriate. If syncope occurs in the setting of documented orthostatic hypotension, then this diagnosis can be made with certainty. If EKG evidence of ischemia, infarct, or an arrhythmia accompanies the syncopal spell, these conditions can be accurately diagnosed. In each of these instances, further testing is not usually necessary.

If the history, physical exam, and EKG are suggestive of the cause, but not certain, than specific testing for the suspected etiology is indicated. For instance, an 85-year-old man may present with syncope and a grade 3/6 systolic murmur that radiates to the carotids. It is suspected that he has aortic stenosis, so an echocardiogram would be appropriately ordered to confirm the suspicion.

If, however, a thorough history, physical exam, and EKG are performed and syncope remains unexplained, then it is important to determine whether the patient has underlying heart disease. The presence of underlying heart disease is the only independent risk factor of a cardiac etiology of syncope. Additionally, in patients with underlying heart disease, syncope is often a warning sign of impending cardiac arrest.

If the patient has no history of heart disease, an echocardiogram and exercise treadmill test may identify occult heart disease. If the patient has reached 60 years of age, has an abnormal EKG, or has symptoms worrisome for underlying heart disease, then these studies are mandatory in unexplained syncope. Symptoms that warrant evaluation for occult heart disease include sudden syncope and exertional symptoms such as chest pain, dyspnea, or syncope. In patients who are 60 and older who don't have these features, it is acceptable to perform carotid sinus massage to exclude carotid sinus hypersensitivity prior to undergoing a cardiac evaluation.

If the echocardiogram and the exercise treadmill reveal no signs of occult heart disease and the patient has had only one episode of syncope, no further workup is indicated. If the

> **Bottom Line**
> If syncope remains unexplained after your initial H&P and EKG, order an echo and treadmill to look for underlying heart disease. If underlying heart disease is present, then evaluate for an arrhythmia either with inpatient telemetry or outpatient Holter monitoring. If this remains nondiagnostic, then consider an electrophysiology study. In young people with no suspicion for cardiac or neurological disease, begin your workup with a tilt table test.

patient has had previous episodes of syncope, then a tilt table test, psychiatric evaluation, or a 30-day monitor may be considered.

If heart disease is identified by the echocardiogram and/or the exercise treadmill, the patient may indeed have a significant arrhythmia. If the patient is being treated as an inpatient, telemetry monitoring may identify an arrhythmia. If the patient is being evaluated as an outpatient, then a Holter monitor is indicated. If the Holter monitor reveals that syncopal spells are accompanied by benign rhythms, then the patient should be evaluated for other causes of syncope. If a malignant arrhythmia is identified, it should be treated appropriately. If the study is nondiagnostic, consider electrophysiology (EP) testing.

Patients with unexplained syncope with no suspected heart disease or a negative EP study, who have had more than one episode may require a tilt table test, psychiatric evaluation, or an event monitor.

In young patients with recurrent syncope and no suspicion of cardiac or neurological disease, tilt testing is recommended for initial workup.

Specific Diagnostic Tests

> **Pearl**
>
> In patients with a BBB on their EKG, syncope is often due to prolonged asystolic pauses.

An EKG is essential during the initial evaluation of syncope. Examples of EKG abnormalities that suggest an arrhythmic etiology of syncope include any conduction abnormalities such as a BBB, widened QRS complex, or Mobitz type II AV block. Presence of Q waves, a prolonged QT interval, or sinus bradycardia are also suggestive of an arrhythmic cause of syncope.

Laboratory studies that may be helpful in the evaluation of syncope include a blood sugar level to assess for hypoglycemia, a CBC to rule out sepsis or hemorrhage, and an electrolyte panel including a magnesium level because electrolyte abnormalities such as hypokalemia can cause arrhythmias.

Carotid sinus massage may reveal carotid sinus hypersensitivity. This test is contraindicated in patients with a carotid bruit, previous CVA, significant carotid artery disease, or previous MI (within 3 months). In order to perform this test, you must first listen for carotid bruits. If no bruits are audible, arrange to have continuous EKG monitoring and blood pressure measurements during the procedure. Next, massage the carotid arterial pulse just below the thyroid cartilage for 5 to 10 seconds. (Never massage both carotid arteries at the same time.) The test is positive if the patient's symptoms are reproduced in conjunction with a blood pressure drop of 50 mmHg or more or if the patient develops 3 or more seconds of asystole.

Tilt table testing is useful in identifying neurocardiogenic syncope. It should be utilized in patients who present with recurrent episodes of syncope but have no underlying heart disease, in patients with heart disease who have had a benign investigation for cardiac causes, and in patients with an unexplained episode of syncope that caused or could have caused substantial harm (for example, in patients who drive a school bus). Tilt testing may also be considered in the evaluation of patients with dizziness, presyncope, or recurrent falls.

An echocardiogram and an exercise treadmill test may detect underlying heart disease and will help guide your decision making. An echocardiogram can be diagnostic if aortic stenosis or hypertrophic obstructive cardiomyopathy is the cause of syncope. Stress testing may be particularly helpful in patients with exertional syncope or if exercise-induced arrhythmias occur.

A 24-hour monitor (Holter or ambulatory monitor) may detect an arrhythmia, but is only useful if the patient has an episode during the time period when the monitor is worn. If patients do not have symptoms or occurrences on a daily basis, it may be beneficial to order a 30-day monitor (event or loop monitor) instead. Patients who have rare symptoms may require an implantable loop recorder. These devices are implanted like a pacemaker and can remain in place for many months to capture a rhythm disturbance during rare cases of syncope.

Neurological studies such as an electroencephalogram may be useful if it is believed that the patient may have actually had a seizure rather than a syncopal spell. A carotid Doppler, head CT scan, or MRI may be obtained if a CVA is suspected.

BACK TO THE BASICS

When under stress, the sympathetic nervous system is activated. This increases the heart rate in anticipation of the need to escape a dangerous situation. It has been suggested that receptors in the heart detect this sympathetic response and attempt to counter this response by stimulating the vagus nerve. The vagus nerve is responsible for stimulating the parasympathetic nervous system resulting in a sudden, dramatic drop in blood pressure and pulse, causing a syncopal spell.

When undergoing a tilt table test, patients are placed in an upright position long enough to allow the blood to pool in their lower extremities. The reduced venous return to the heart stimulates the heart to beat faster to provide more oxygen to the tissues. In patients with vasovagal syncope, the vagus is stimulated by this increase in heart rate, resulting in a dramatic reduction in blood pressure and pulse. A loss of postural tone or frank syncope will be observed. Simply returning the patient to a recumbent or Trendelenburg position alleviates the venous pooling and allows the patient to recover.

Management

Management is directed at the underlying cause of syncope. Presyncope and dizziness, the prodromal symptoms of frank syncope, are managed in much the same way as syncope.

To Admit or Not to Admit?

Admission may be considered if patients are elderly, have sustained serious injury, or are suspected to have a serious cardiovascular or neurological condition precipitating the syncopal spells.

Cardio Reality

Mrs. H is a 65-year-old woman whom I was asked to see in consultation for syncope. When I arrived at her bedside, I observed that she had sustained significant trauma. Despite the bandages, I could see that she was bruised and battered. I introduced myself, asked her how she was doing, and then began to obtain a history.

Mrs. H was a previously healthy woman who had been driving her car down a street in a large city. The next thing she knew, she was being assisted out of her car, which was situated in the front room of a beauty parlor. She was surprised to learn that she had driven her car through the front glass window. She recalled no prodromal symptoms, had no loss of bowel or bladder continence, and had no prior history of cardiovascular disease, seizures, strokes, or prior episodes of syncope. She specifically denied any chest pain, dyspnea, palpitations, dizziness, or visual changes just prior to the event, subsequent to the event, or over the past few months. Despite her injuries, she felt fine after being escorted out of the car, and denied any confusion, slurred speech, or weakness of any extremities.

Other than her obvious trauma, her physical exam was benign including carotid sinus massage. The CBC, BMP, cardiac enzymes, drug screen, EKG, and CXR from the ED were all within normal limits.

Given the sudden nature of her syncope, a cardiac evaluation was essential. The patient was already on telemetry and an echocardiogram and an ischemic evaluation with a treadmill stress test was ordered. (She claimed she was well enough to perform one.)

Prior to undergoing her studies, the patient developed an episode of ventricular tachycardia that was captured on telemetry and the etiology of her syncope was identified.

Mrs. H's history of sudden syncope revealed the serious nature of her syncope and resulted in a careful cardiac evaluation, including telemetry monitoring. Be sure to perform a detailed history and physical on all patients with syncope.

What About Driving Privileges?

If the patient experiences warning symptoms, can avoid the known precipitating causes, and has infrequent episodes of syncope, then driving restrictions may not be as stringent.

If, however, patients have unpredictable symptoms or syncope is not controlled despite appropriate management of the underlying condition, then driving cessation is recommended. In neurocardiogenic syncope, use your clinical judgment based on the severity of the presenting event and precipitating factors.

Chapter 15

Palpitations

Introduction

Palpitations are an unpleasant awareness of one's heartbeat. Patients may describe these as "racing," "fluttering," "skipping," or an "electric sensation." Ask the patient to tap out the rhythm to get a better idea of what they are describing.

Differential Diagnosis

Cardiac causes are the most common etiology of palpitations in patients who present to the ED, while psychiatric causes are more common when patients present to outpatient clinics.

Cardiac causes include arrhythmias, valvular heart disease, atrial myxomas, cardiomyopathy. Inappropriate sinus tachycardia, a rare disorder that results in a fast heart rate with minimal exertion or emotional stress, may also cause palpitations.

Psychiatric causes include panic attacks, anxiety disorders, somatization, and depression. When treating patients with a psychiatric history, be careful not to assume that palpitations are due to the underlying psychiatric condition without considering alternative, possibly life-threatening, etiologies.

Other disorders that may cause palpitations include hypoglycemia, thyrotoxicosis, pheochromocytoma, anemia, pregnancy, and fever. Increased catecholamine production during stress and exercise may lead to palpitations.

Bronchodilators, anticholinergics, sympathomimetics, and vasodilators are examples of medications that may cause palpitations, as may cocaine, amphetamines, alcohol, nicotine, and caffeine. Palpitations may also occur when patients discontinue beta-blockers.

Historical Questions to Narrow Your Differential

When Did You First Notice the Palpitations? Do You Recall Having Similar Episodes in the Past?

Patients who have had rapid palpitations on and off throughout life may have AV-nodal reentrant tachycardia or a supraventricular tachycardia (SVT) that utilizes a bypass tract.

Atrial fibrillation or atrial tachycardia, on the other hand, are more commonly associated with onset in advanced age.

Can You Describe the Palpitations? Do They Feel Like a Flip-Flop, Racing, Fluttering, or Pounding in the Neck? Can You Tap Out the Rhythm for Me?

A rapid and regular rhythm is more likely due to an SVT, while a rapid irregular rhythm is more likely due to atrial fibrillation or a tachycardia with variable blocking through the AV node as may occur in atrial flutter.

Patients with premature contractions such as PVCs often describe a sensation of a long pause followed by a loud thump. This "flip-flopping" indicates the compensatory pause after a premature contraction followed by the subsequent normal beat. Because the premature beat often is inefficient and does not eject the full volume of blood, there will be an increased volume of blood to pump in the subsequent, normally conducted, beat. This increased volume results in the perceived loud thump.

Rapid fluttering may signify a sustained sinus tachycardia, supraventricular, or ventricular rhythm.

When the atrium contracts against a closed mitral or tricuspid valve, patients may complain of a pounding sensation in their neck. This occurs when the atria and ventricles are beating independently of one another as in complete heart block.

Do the Palpitations Come On Gradually or Suddenly? Do They End Gradually or Suddenly?

A gradual start and stop is commonly associated with sinus tachycardia while abrupt onset and offset are common signs of a supraventricular or ventricular tachycardia. Patients may say that their heart "just took off."

If patients can terminate their palpitations with carotid sinus massage or Valsalva maneuvers, they are most likely AV reentrant tachycardia or an SVT with a bypass tract.

Are the Palpitations Accompanied by Any Other Symptoms?

Palpitations accompanied by dizziness or syncope are more ominous and warrant an immediate evaluation for a potentially life-threatening arrhythmia.

Do You Notice These Palpitations When You Have a Caffeinated Product? Have You Been Taking Any OTC Cold Medicines or Using Alcohol, Tobacco, or Illicit Drugs?

These substances may precipitate palpitations and you should inquire about their use.

Are You Under Any Significant Stress?

Stress can precipitate palpitations.

What Other Medical Problems Do You Have and What Medications Are You Taking?

Be sure to inquire about symptoms related to hypoglycemia, thyrotoxicosis, and pheochromocytoma. Inquire about any history of cardiac or psychiatric conditions.

Bottom Line

I have included references to reentrant tachycardias, bypass tracts, and other very advanced concepts here for the sake of completeness and for the benefit of our seasoned cardiovascular specialty readers. Please don't be overwhelmed if you are not familiar with these rhythms, the workup is still the same! Simply try to capture the arrhythmia on a monitor and a cardiologist or electrophysiologist can determine if any of these more advanced arrhythmias are present and then decide how to manage it.

Physical Exam

A complete physical exam will be helpful in identifying both the cardiac and noncardiac disorders that may be causing palpitations. Pay particularly close attention to the cardiac exam because you would not want to miss a life-threatening cardiac cause.

Diagnostic Strategy and Management

A CBC, chemistry panel, and thyroid function tests are essential to rule out metabolic dyscrasias, which may contribute to palpitations.

A 12-lead EKG may reveal a dysrhythmia if the patient is currently symptomatic. You may also discover signs of ischemia, hypertensive heart disease, or preexcitation syndromes.

A 24-hour ambulatory monitor (Holter monitor) may identify the cause of intermittent palpitations, provided they occur during the 24-hour period when you are monitoring. If symptoms occur less frequently, a 30-day monitor may be required. It is useful to have the patient keep a diary of symptoms during the monitoring period so that you can correlate their perception of symptoms with the rhythm detected on the monitor. This is useful in reassuring patients who have benign arrhythmias.

Management is geared toward the underlying cause. Additionally, you should educate the patient about anything that may be precipitating the attacks such as wearing tight collars in carotid sinus hypersensitivity. Instruct the patient to avoid substances that may aggravate symptoms such as alcohol, tobacco, caffeine, OTC cold preparations, and stress.

Chapter 16

Edema

Introduction

Edema occurs when fluid moves from the vascular space to the interstitial space. This may occur because the capillaries have increased permeability, decreased oncotic pressure, or increased hydrostatic pressure. Obstruction of the lymphatic circulation, due to surgical excision of lymph nodes or malignancies that obstruct the lymphatic system, may also cause edema.

BACK TO THE BASICS

Capillary permeability increases when the capillary wall is damaged or the pores are enlarged. This may occur in burns or tissue damage or in allergic reactions or inflammation. Malignancies can also cause increased capillary permeability as seen when these patients develop pleural effusions or ascites.

A reduction of osmotic pressure may occur if less protein exists as in malnutrition or starvation. Because the liver produces protein, hepatic impairment also results in decreased protein in circulation. Increased loss of protein due to extensive burns or proteinuria, which accompanies certain renal diseases, also reduces the osmotic pressure.

Increased hydrostatic pressure may occur if the vascular volume is increased. Conditions that increase the vascular volume include pregnancy, premenstrual syndrome (PMS), CHF, and renal disease. Venous obstruction, as in thrombophlebitis or portal hypertension due to liver disease, also causes increased hydrostatic pressure.

(continues)

> ## BACK TO THE BASICS (continued)
>
> In order to return to the heart, the blood must first pass through the liver. In severe liver disease, the blood may not be able to pass through the liver. This causes a backup of fluid behind the liver. Because the heart is continuously pumping blood forward but there is some obstruction prohibiting the blood from passing the liver, there is increased hydrostatic pressure ("hydro" meaning water or fluid and "static" meaning still). Essentially the fluid can not go anywhere, so it is sitting still. The heart keeps pumping more blood, thereby forcing it to go somewhere, so it is squeezed out of the bloodstream and into the interstitial space, causing edema.
>
> The kidneys are responsible for retaining sodium and water when necessary to achieve homeostasis. When there is increased movement of fluid from the vasculature to the interstitial space, the kidneys begin to retain more sodium and water in an effort to replete the vascular volume and avoid shock. This results in a further increase in the vascular volume and, therefore, worsening edema.

Differential Diagnosis

The three organ systems most likely to cause edema when impaired are the cardiovascular, hepatic, or renal systems. Some clues that help distinguish between these etiologies include whether pulmonary edema is present and whether the JVP is elevated.

When pulmonary edema exists, the most likely etiology is cardiac disease. If a patient presents with acute pulmonary edema, be sure to rule out an underlying acute MI.

Pulmonary edema can also result from acute glomerulonephritis, because increased sodium retention by the kidneys leads to volume overload, or acute respiratory distress syndrome (RDS) due to increased capillary permeability.

> **Pearl**
>
> Pulmonary edema should be considered a sign of an acute MI until proven otherwise.

The JVP will be elevated in patients with an increased volume of fluid in circulation, such as in sodium retention from renal disease. Right ventricular heart failure also results in an elevated JVP because the blood backs up behind the right side of the heart into the vena cava and subsequently to the neck veins. The JVP will not be elevated in cirrhosis or hepatic disease. This is because the circulation is obstructed at the liver, and fluid only backs up below the liver.

The classic tetrad of edema, severe protein-uria, hypoalbuminemia, and hyperlipidemia, indicates nephrotic syndrome. The renal impairment in nephrotic syndrome results in sodium retention and therefore volume expansion. This expanded fluid volume would normally be expected to increase the JVP. However, decreased oncotic pressure because of hypoalbuminemia causes leaking of the volume into the interstitium. This leaking of fluid volume lowers the JVP, resulting in a net JVP that is either normal or high normal.

> **Bottom Line**
> If pulmonary edema is present, consider a cardiac cause. Other possibilities include glomerulonephritis or respiratory distress syndrome.

Venous insufficiency is a common cause of peripheral edema. It may occur acutely after an episode of thrombophlebitis or it may be chronic due to poor functioning of the valves in the veins associated with aging. (The valves in the veins prevent blood from flowing in the wrong direction.) Venous insufficiency only affects the lower extremities so there will be no pulmonary edema or elevation of JVP.

> **Bottom Line**
> If the JVP is elevated, consider a renal or cardiac etiology of edema. If the JVP is normal, consider hepatic disease, venous insufficiency, or other causes.

Unilateral peripheral edema may be a result of venous insufficiency, but take care to exclude deep vein thrombosis (DVT).

Nonpitting edema may occur in pretibial myxedema of thyroid disease or in chronic venous stasis. Lymphedema, which may be a result of lymphatic disease or removal of the lymph nodes as in a radical mastectomy, may also result in nonpitting edema.

Any local injury can cause edema; patients who have had a saphenous vein graft often have subsequent edema of the extremity from which the graft was harvested.

Edema may simply be the result of an adverse drug reaction. The dihydropyridine CCBs (such as amlodipine) commonly cause edema particularly at higher dosages.

Historical Questions to Narrow Your Differential

Where Is the Edema Located?

Anasarca is generalized edema that may result from severe heart failure, cirrhosis, or nephrotic syndrome. Superior vena cava syndrome, which may indicate carcinoma of the lung, results in edema of the face, arms, and neck.

Abdominal edema (ascites) may be due to cirrhosis. Peripheral edema may be due to heart failure, a renal disorder, or local venous disease.

Is the Edema Intermittent or Persistent?

Some women will have intermittent edema due to PMS. Poor compliance with sodium restriction may result in intermittent exacerbations of edema.

Does the Patient Have a History of, or Symptoms Associated with, a Cardiac, Hepatic, or Renal Disorder?

Cardiac causes are the most common cause of pedal edema if pulmonary edema is also present. Patients with pulmonary edema may complain of exertional dyspnea, orthopnea, or PND. If no symptoms are present, you may hear rales on the lung exam. Edema of cardiac origin that is not accompanied by dyspnea or orthopnea suggests a right-sided heart lesion such as tricuspid stenosis. An echocardiogram will help identify a right-sided lesion.

Symptoms of hepatic impairment include jaundice, fatigue, pruritus, and abdominal distention. Liver function studies will assist in making the diagnosis.

Uremia, the clinical syndrome that results from renal failure, may present with nausea, vomiting, pruritus, fatigue, anorexia, weight loss, muscle cramps, and altered mental status. Serum BUN and creatinine levels will help distinguish these nonspecific findings from other disorders.

Is the Patient on Any Medications that May Cause Cardiac, Hepatic, or Renal Impairment?

The glitazones may cause heart failure by increasing vascular volume. NSAIDS, ACE inhibitors, gentamycin, and vancomycin are all nephrotoxic. Methotrexate and isoniazid (INH) are hepatotoxic.

Physical Exam

General: Note the patient's skin tone. Uremia, a subtle pale-yellowish color, may be evident in renal disease. Jaundice may be present in hepatic disease.

Skin: Spider nevi may be present in hepatic impairment.

HEENT: Periorbital edema may occur in nephrotic syndrome. Inspect the conjunctiva for icterus (yellow discoloration), which may indicate hepatic disease.

Neck: Assess the JVP.

Lungs: Auscultate the lungs for rales. Gynecomastia may be observed during your lung exam and is often present in hepatic disorders.

Heart: Palpate for the PMI. Listen for heart murmurs or extra sounds.
Abdomen: Assess the abdomen for signs of ascites (fluid wave, shifting dullness) or hepatomegaly.
Extremities: Assess for peripheral edema. Remember to check dependent areas. If the patient is bedridden, fluid may accumulate in the sacrum rather than the lower extremities. Some men will develop scrotal edema, which can be profound and particularly unsettling for the patient. Assess whether the edema is pitting or nonpitting by pressing your finger on the edematous area. Remember that edema can be tender.

Assess the lower extremities for signs of venous insufficiency: brownish "brawny" discoloration around the ankles, thickening of the skin, and ulcers around the medial malleolus.

If unilateral edema is suspected, confirm by measuring the circumference of the legs. Calf tenderness, a palpable cord, and/or a positive Homan's sign suggest the possibility of an underlying DVT. A positive Homan's sign occurs when the patient develops pain in their calf with forcible dorsiflexion of the ankle while the knee is flexed.

Neuro: Assess for asterixis if hepatic disease is suspected. Ask the patient to hold their arms forward with their hands flexed upright with the fingers spread. Sudden nonrhythmic flexion of the hands and fingers is indicative of asterixis.

Diagnostic Strategy and Management

Use your clinical judgment to decide which studies are needed after conducting a thorough history and physical exam. Some studies you may wish to order include liver function tests and/or a PT/INR to assess hepatic function, serum BUN and creatinine to assess renal function, and a CBC to assess for anemia, which is often associated with renal failure and can lead to heart failure. A plasma albumin level and thyroid function studies may also be indicated.

Diuretics are useful in generalized edema as with heart failure, nephritic syndrome, and primary sodium retention. Loop diuretics such as furosemide (Lasix) are considered first line except in cirrhosis where spironolactone is considered first line.

When using diuretics, the plasma BUN and creatinine should be monitored to ensure that the plasma volume has not diminished too much leading to poor perfusion of the kidneys and other vital organs. Fatigue, weakness, orthostatic dizziness, and confusion may occur if overdiuresis leads to decreased cerebral blood flow.

Patients with edema due to venous insufficiency should avoid diuretics or use them with caution, because they will deplete the plasma volume. These patients do not have excess fluid volume requiring diuresis; rather, they need to redirect the fluid back to where it belongs. Support stockings, contraction of the leg musculature (as with movement), and elevation of the extremities above the heart all serve this purpose.

Lymphedema is more difficult to treat. Compression garments and massage therapy may be considered.

SECTION III RESOURCES

Baliga, Ragavendra, Anjana Siva, and Mark Noble, 2005. *Crash Course: Cardiology.* Philadelphia, PA: Elsevier Mosby.

Bickley, Lynn S. *Bates' Guide to Physical Examination and History Taking,* 8th ed. 2003. Philadelphia, PA: Lippincott Williams & Wilkins.

Cavley Jr., William E. "Diagnosing the Cause of Chest Pain." *American Family Physician* 72(10):2012.

Crawford, Peter A. and Tammy L. Lin. 2004. *Washington Manual Subspecialty Consult Series: Cardiology Subspecialty Consult.* Philadelphia, PA: Lippincott Williams & Wilkins.

Howes, David, and Ethan Booker. 2005. *Myocarditis.* Retrieved from www.emedicine.com/ EMERG/topic326.htm. Accessed November 25, 2006.

Karnath, Bernard, Mark Holden, and Nassir Hussain. 2004. "Chest Pain: Differentiating Cardiac from Noncardiac Pain." *Hospital Physician* 40(4): 24–27, 38.

Kasper, Braunwald, Fauci, et al. 2005. *Harrison's Principles of Internal Medicine,* 16th ed. New York, NY: McGraw Hill.

Olshansky, Brian. *Evaluation of the Patient with Syncope.* Retrieved from www.utdol.com. Accessed August 28, 2006.

Physician's Guide to Assessing and Counseling Older Drivers. Retrieved from www.nhtsa.gov/ people/injury/olddrive/OlderDriversBook/pages/Ch9-Section3.html. Accessed August 28, 2006.

Porth, Carol Mattson. 2005. *Pathophysiology: Concepts of Altered Health States,* 7th ed. Philadelphia, PA: Lippincott Williams & Wilkins.

Rose, Burton. *Approach to the Adult with Edema.* Retrieved from www.uptodate.com. Accessed August 21, 2006.

Tierney, L.M., S.J. McPhee, et al. 2005. *Current Medical Diagnosis and Treatment,* 44th ed. New York, NY: Lange.

Topol, Eric J. 2002. *Textbook of Cardiovascular Medicine,* 2nd ed. Philadelphia, PA: Lippincott Williams & Wilkins.

Zimetbaum, Peter J. *Overview of Palpitations.* Retrieved from www.utdol.com. Accessed August 25, 2006.

Cardio Conditions

The role of physician assistants and nurse practitioners is variable depending on the state laws governing their practice, the type of practice in which they are employed, and their relationship with their supervising physician. Despite these differences, certain cardiovascular conditions are certain to be managed frequently by PAs and NPs. The conditions discussed in this section were specifically selected because of the large role that PAs and NPs have in their management. Additionally, topics that are commonly found on certification examinations have been included.

*Most of the management information in this section was adapted from the American College of Cardiology and/or the American Heart Association guidelines. It is wise to keep abreast of new guidelines from these organizations as they are released. This information can be found at **www.americanheart.org** under the heading, "Scientific Statements and Practice Guidelines Topic List."*

Chapter 17

Hypertension and Orthostatic Hypotension

Introduction

Hypertension (HTN) is an important condition for PAs and NPs to treat properly for several reasons. First, it is exceedingly common; approximately 27% of American adults battle with hypertension. Second, it leads to cardiovascular, cerebrovascular, and renal disability. Lastly, we can do something about it; hypertension is a modifiable cardiovascular risk factor.

BACK TO THE BASICS

The stroke volume (SV), which is the amount of blood forced out of the heart with each beat, is determined by preload, afterload, and contractility. Preload is the amount of blood available to be pumped with each beat and is dependent on ventricular filling by venous return to the heart. Afterload is the degree of resistance the heart has to overcome in order to pump the blood forward. The pressure within the aorta determines left ventricular afterload while the pulmonary artery pressure determines the afterload of the right ventricle. Contractility is the intrinsic ability of the heart muscle to pump.

Cardiac output (CO) is the product of the stroke volume and the heart rate (HR). The amount of blood that the heart can circulate depends on the volume pumped out with each beat multiplied by the number of beats per minute. Essentially, if the stroke volume is decreased due to a reduction in intravascular blood volume, so is the cardiac output.

Blood pressure (BP) is the product of cardiac output and total peripheral resistance (TPR). Essentially, blood pressure is a product of the amount of blood circulating and the resistance to flow that is caused by the vessels. HTN can be caused by anything that adversely affects the above.

For Example

Excess sodium intake leads to volume expansion, which increases preload. Increased preload increases the stroke volume, which increases cardiac output, which increases blood pressure.

Bottom Line

SV = preload
× afterload
× contractility
CO = SV × HR
BP = CO × TPR

Classification of Hypertension

The Seventh Report of the Joint National Committee on Prevention, Detection, Evaluation and Treatment of High Blood Pressure has classified the stages of hypertension as follows:

Normal	< 120 systolic and < 80 diastolic
Prehypertension	120–139 systolic or 80–89 diastolic
Stage 1 HTN	140–159 systolic or 90–99 diastolic
Stage 2 HTN	> 159 systolic or > 99 diastolic

Evaluation of HTN

When evaluating a patient with HTN, assess for signs or symptoms of end-organ damage, screen for other cardiac risk factors and comorbidities, and identify possible underlying causes of hypertension. Assess the patient's response to therapy if treatment has already been initiated. A thorough history and physical and several basic tests will help achieve these goals.

History

When performing the HPI, determine when the patient was initially diagnosed with hypertension. Inquire about symptoms that were previously or are currently present. The majority of hypertensive patients are asymptomatic and are diagnosed by routine screening; however, many patients may complain of a throbbing headache in the occipital region. Other possible symptoms include chest pain, dyspnea, tachycardia, claudication, and visual disturbances.

During the PMH, screen for pertinent comorbidities, which include the following:

- CHD
- CHF
- Cerebrovascular disease

- Peripheral vascular disease
- Diabetes mellitus
- Renal disorders
- Sexual dysfunction

Also, inquire about the following risk factors:

- Tobacco smoking
- Excessive alcohol intake
- Sedentary lifestyle
- Dyslipidemia
- Diabetes mellitus (both a comorbidity and a risk factor)

While reviewing the patient's medication list, be sure to specifically inquire about corticosteroids, sympathomimetics (often found in OTC cold medications such as pseudoephedrine), estrogens, caffeine, or any other herbal, homeopathic, or OTC medications.

Determine whether there is a family history of hypertension, pheochromocytoma, renal disorders, diabetes mellitus, or dyslipidemia.

A complete social history should include diet and exercise routines; habits such as smoking, alcohol, or illicit drug use; any stressors; and daily activities.

Physical Examination

When performing a physical examination on a patient with HTN, determine height and weight and calculate their body mass index (BMI) or waist-to-hip ratio. Perform a fundoscopic exam to assess for hypertensive retinopathy, hemorrhage, or exudates. Examine the neck for carotid bruits and thyroid masses or enlargement. Perform a thorough cardiac examination including auscultation of the heart with attention to rate, rhythm, extra heart sounds, or murmurs. Locate the PMI to determine if it has been laterally displaced. Auscultate the lungs for adventitious sounds. Auscultate for aortic or renal bruits. Palpate peripheral pulses and inspect and palpate for edema. Perform a neurological examination with attention to possible signs of a previous stroke.

Diagnostic Studies

During the initial evaluation of HTN, the following studies should be performed:

- Urinalysis to identify renal disease
- Basic metabolic panel to assess for low potassium (as in hyperaldosteronism), elevated glucose (as in diabetes), and elevated blood urea nitrogen and creatinine (as in renal disease)

- Complete blood cell count to identify possible polycythemia, which can cause secondary hypertension
- Lipid panel for risk stratification
- Electrocardiogram to identify coronary heart disease or left ventricular hypertrophy

---

Bottom Line

Initial workup of HTN should include a thorough H&P along with an EKG, U/A, serum glucose, hematocrit, electrolytes, serum creatinine, and a lipid panel.

Management of HTN

Patients with HTN should be treated to a target BP of 140/90 mmHg or less. In patients with diabetes or chronic kidney disease, the target is reduced to 130/80 mmHg or less. Lifestyle modifications should be instituted first or along with medications.

Lifestyle Modifications

Lifestyle modifications include weight reduction, sodium restriction, aerobic exercise, and moderation of alcohol consumption. The DASH diet has been proven to lower blood pressure in patients with prehypertension and stage 1 hypertension. It emphasizes fruits, vegetables, and low-fat diary products. It also includes increased fiber, whole grains, poultry, and nuts. It encourages less red meat, sweets, and sugared drinks. The DASH diet results in reduced total fat, saturated fat, cholesterol, and sodium.

Antihypertensive Medications

If the patient has no compelling indications, choose a thiazide diuretic, ACE inhibitor, ARB, beta-blocker, or CCB for stage 1 hypertensive patients. For stage 2 hypertensive patients, choose a combination product such as the CCB/ACE inhibitor combination (Lotrel) or an ACEI or ARB in combination with a diuretic. If the initial medication does not reduce the patient's BP to goal, optimize the dose or add additional drugs. The majority of patients require more than one antihypertensive agent to reach their BP goal.

There are several classes of medications for hypertension. The diuretics include the thiazides such as hydrochlorothiazide (HCTZ) and chlorthalidone and the loop diuretics such as furosemide (Lasix), torsemide (Demadex), and bumetanide (Bumex).

The CCBs include the dihydropyridines such as amlodipine (Norvasc), isradipine (Dynacirc CR), nifedipine XL, and the nondihydropyridines such as verapamil and diltiazem.

The adrenergic inhibitors include the beta-blockers, (i.e., metoprolol [Toprol XL], atenolol [Tenormin], and propranolol [Inderal]), the alpha- and beta-receptor blockers (i.e., labetalol [Trandate] and carvedilol [Coreg]), the centrally acting agents such as clonidine (Catapres) and methyldopa (Aldomet), and the alpha-receptor blockers such as doxazosin (Cardura) and terazosin (Hytrin).

ACE inhibitors include lisinopril (Prinivil, Zestril), benazepril (Lotensin), captopril (Capoten), enalapril (Vasotec), fosinopril (Monopril), moexipril (Univasc), quinapril (Accupril), ramipril (Altace), and trandolapril (Aceon).

ARBs include valsartan (Diovan), candesartan (Atacand), telmisartan (Micardis), olmesartan (Benicar), losartan (Cozaar), irbesartan (Avapro), and eprosartan (Teveten).

The aldosterone antagonists include spironolactone (Aldactone) and eplerenone (Inspra).

The direct vasodilators include hydralazine and minoxidil.

Tekturna (aliskiren) is the first of a new class of medications called renin inhibitors. It was released in March of 2007.

Compelling Indications

If the patient has a compelling indication for a particular antihypertensive, select that medication first. Compelling indications and their recommended medications include the following:

- Heart failure: beta-blockers, ACE inhibitors, ARBs, aldosterone antagonists, or thiazide diuretics
- Post-MI: beta-blockers, ACE inhibitors, aldosterone antagonists
- High risk of cardiovascular disease: beta-blockers, ACE inhibitors, CCBs, or thiazide diuretics
- Diabetes: ACE inhibitors, ARBs, beta-blockers, CCBs, thiazide diuretics *
- Chronic kidney disease: ACE inhibitors or ARBs
- Recurrent stroke prevention: ACE inhibitors or thiazide diuretics

---

* Most beta-blockers and higher doses of thiazide diuretics (i.e., 25 mg/day hydrochlorothiazide) are known to worsen insulin resistance, thereby increasing the risk of developing diabetes. This effect has not been seen with the use of CCBs or ACE inhibitors. Whether the increased incidence of diabetes worsens cardiovascular endpoints is not yet known. For this reason, increased monitoring for the development of diabetes is suggested for patients taking beta-blockers and/or thiazide diuretics. Consider using the ACEI/CCB combination product, Lotrel, in lieu of an ACEI or ARB in combination with a diuretic if this is a concern.

Diagnosing Secondary Hypertension

Secondary HTN results from an identifiable underlying cause. Essential HTN, where no identifiable cause can be elicited, is far more common and accounts for 90–95% of hypertensives.

Suspect a secondary cause if the patient is over the age of 50 or under the age of 20 (under the age of 30 if the patient is nonobese, nonblack and has no family history of HTN) at the time of onset of HTN. Also, suspect a secondary cause if the patient has poor response to therapy or develops worsening control of their blood pressure, has significantly elevated BP (SBP > 180 mmHg or DSP > 110 mmHg), or significant end-organ damage.

Secondary HTN may be due to sleep apnea, chronic kidney disease, primary aldosteronism, renovascular disease, Cushings syndrome or steroid use, pheochromocytoma, coarctation of the aorta, or thyroid/parathyroid disease.

Secondary hypertension may also be drug induced. The following are examples of drugs that may raise the blood pressure:

- Immunosuppressive agents
- NSAIDs
- COX-2 inhibitors
- Estrogens
- Weight loss agents such as ephedra or sibutramine (Meridia)
- Stimulants such as amphetamines or nicotine
- Mineralocorticoids such as fludrocortisone (Florinef)
- Antiparkinsonian drugs such as bromocriptine (Parlodel)
- MAO inhibitors
- Anabolic steroids
- Sympathomimetics such as pseudoephedrine (Sudafed)

When performing your H&P, be on the lookout for clues that suggest a secondary cause. For instance, snoring, daytime somnolence, and obesity suggest sleep apnea; order a sleep study. An abdominal bruit may suggest renovascular disease; order an MRA, captopril renal scan, or renal arteriography. Diminished femoral pulses may indicate coarctation of the aorta; a CXR and CT of the aorta will help identify this condition. Weight gain, moon facies, hirsutism, truncal obesity, striae, a buffalo hump, and amenorrhea suggest Cushing's syndrome; order a dexamethasone suppression test. Episodic HTN with a headache, palpitations, tachycardia, and diaphoresis suggest the possibility of a pheochromocytoma; order a 24-hour urine for vanillylmandelic acid (VMA), metanephrines, and normetanephrines and plasma-free metanephrines. Consider hyperthyroidism if heat intolerance, weight loss, palpitations, exophthalmos, tremor, and tachycardia are present; order a TSH level. If kidney stones, osteoporosis, depression, lethargy, and muscle weakness are present, consider hyperparathyroidism and order serum calcium and parathyroid hormone levels.

When reviewing your initial labwork, secondary causes of HTN may be revealed. If you identify hypernatremia and hypokalemia that is not caused by diuretic use, order a ratio of plasma aldosterone levels to plasma renin activity and CT scan of the adrenals to diagnose aldosteronism. If you uncover renal insufficiency and proteinuria, consider the possibility of renal parenchymal disease; order a renal ultrasound.

Bottom Line

ABCDE mnemonic for Secondary Causes of HTN:

A: **A**ccuracy of diagnosis, obstructive sleep **A**pnea, **A**ldosteronism

B: renal artery **B**ruits (suggests renal artery stenosis), **B**ad kidneys (renal parenchymal disease)

C: excess **C**atecholamines, **C**oarctation of the aorta, **C**ushing's syndrome

D: **D**rugs, **D**iet

E: excess **E**rythropoietin, **E**ndocrine disorders

Complications

Complications of HTN include heart disease, cerebrovascular disease, and renal disease. Arterial damage such as aneurysm formation and large vessel disease such as abdominal aortic aneurysm or aortic dissection may also result.

Isolated Systolic HTN

Isolated systolic hypertension is defined as a systolic BP greater than or equal to 140 mmHg with a diastolic blood pressure less than 90 mmHg. It is caused by the reduced elasticity of arteries that accompanies aging. Diuretics are helpful in treating this type of hypertension.

Pearl

If you struggle with the fundoscopic exam, consider trying the newer panoptic ophthalmoscopes or ask another provider to take a look with you.

Hypertensive Crises

Although fairly uncommon, hypertensive crises can be life threatening. Hypertensive crises include hypertensive urgencies, emergencies, and pseudo-emergencies.

When a patient presents with elevated blood pressure, inquire about symptoms of chest pain, dyspnea, headache, visual changes, seizures, or other neurological symptoms such as altered mental status. These are all symptoms that may suggest end-organ damage. Ensure all medications are being taken correctly and inquire about any OTC medications or any illicit drugs that may have elevated the BP.

Your physical exam should focus on whether end-organ damage is present. A fundoscopic exam is essential to look for papilledema, exudates, or hemorrhages. Perform a complete cardiac exam with attention to any heart failure signs and perform a neurologic exam.

Order a CBC, BMP, UA, ECG, and a chest radiograph. Order a head CT if a CVA is suspected. If an MI is in the differential, order serial cardiac enzymes.

Management involves lowering the blood pressure. How urgently this needs to be accomplished depends on whether end-organ damage is present.

Hypertensive Urgency

Hypertensive urgencies are severe elevations of BP, but without signs of end-organ damage. Most of these patients are nonadherent to drug therapy or are inadequately treated hypertensive patients who may arrive at the office for other reasons. These patients may also develop HTN as a postoperative complication.

The goal in hypertensive urgencies is to lower the blood pressure no more than 20% over the first several hours. These patients can be discharged with plans to decrease BP over several hours or days. Simply arrange follow-up within 24 hours to several days depending on the individual characteristics of the patient. Of course, be sure the patient is aware of symptoms of end-organ damage and knows how to act immediately should these symptoms arise. Treatment options include:

- Clonidine 0.1 mg po every hour until goal BP is achieved.
- Labetalol 100mg po BID with titration to reach goal BP.

Do *not* use short-acting CCBs such as nifedipine, which may result in decreased cerebral perfusion, hypotension, and myocardial ischemia or infarct.

Hypertensive Emergency

A hypertensive emergency is when elevated blood pressure results in end-organ damage. These are emergency situations that require intensive care (ICU) monitoring and the use of parenteral medications to lower the blood pressure immediately. Both malignant hypertension and hypertensive encephalopathy are examples of hypertensive emergencies.

Malignant Hypertension

Malignant hypertension is the term used for elevated BP that is associated with renal failure, retinopathy, or other end-organ damage. Examples include intracranial hemorrhage, unstable angina pectoris, acute myocardial infarction, acute left ventricular failure with pulmonary edema, aortic dissection, or eclampsia.

The patient's BP is usually, *but not always,* very high (greater than 180/120 mmHg). The presentation may include headache, restlessness, confusion, stupor, motor and/or sensory deficits, or visual disturbances. In severe cases, the patient may present with convulsions or in a coma. Diastolic BP greater than 120 mmHg is typical.

Management includes continuous BP monitoring in the ICU with immediate reduction of BP (within minutes)—however, be careful to avoid excessively rapid BP lowering, which may worsen end-organ damage. As a rule of thumb, aim for a diastolic blood pressure of 100–110 in the first few minutes to hours and do not lower the mean arterial blood pressure more than 25% in the first few hours. An exception is in patients with aortic dissection, LV failure, or pulmonary edema; these patients should have their BP lowered rapidly.

Treatment options include:

- Sodium nitroprusside 0.25 μg/kg/min IV with titration every 5 minutes to a maximum dose of 10 μg/kg/min until goal BP is attained. Sodium nitroprusside may increase intracranial pressure and may cause thiocyanate toxicity. Measure levels if continued for more than 24 hours. Symptoms of thiocyanate toxicity include nausea, anorexia, headache, and/or mental status changes.
- Labetalol 20–40 mg IV bolus every 10–15 minutes or IV infusion of 0.5–2 mg/min. Labetalol can be used in aortic dissection or eclampsia, but is contraindicated in heart failure, AV block, bradycardia, and COPD.
- NTG 5–15 ug/min IV infusion. NTG is an excellent choice in MI, ischemia, or pulmonary edema.
- Hydralazine 10–20 mg IV. Avoid hydralazine in aortic dissection, MI, or ischemia.

Hypertensive Encephalopathy

Hypertensive encephalopathy is a sudden and marked increase in BP that results in cerebral edema. Patients may present with a severe headache, vision changes, seizures, mental status changes, or other neurologic symptoms. On physical exam, you may observe papilledema.

This is reversible with a rapid lowering of BP. Shoot for a 20% reduction in the mean arterial pressure or a diastolic BP of 100 (whichever is the greater reduction) within an hour. Treatment options include:

- Sodium nitroprusside 0.25 µg/kg/min IV with titration every 5 minutes to a maximum dose of 10 µg/kg/min until goal BP is attained.
- Labetalol 20–40 mg IV bolus every 10–15 minutes or IV infusion of 0.5–2 mg/min. Avoid the use of CNS depressants such as clonidine in these patients.

Aortic Dissection

An *aortic aneurysm* is an expandable outpouching of the aorta that is caused by a weakening of the wall. HTN is an important risk factor for the development of an aortic aneurysm, but congenital bicuspid aortic valves, pregnancy, and connective tissue diseases such as Marfan's syndrome may also predispose patients to an aortic aneurysm.

An aortic aneurysm may lead to an aortic dissection if a tear develops in the intima allowing a false channel to form. Type A aortic dissections involve the ascending aorta and are managed with emergent surgery. Type B aortic dissections involve the descending aorta and are typically medically managed with antihypertensives due to the high operative mortality rate. Labetalol or esmolol are good choices for initial therapy because they will lower the heart rate; either agent can then be followed by sodium nitroprusside.

Pseudoemergencies

Pseudoemergencies occur when an underlying condition that causes massive sympathetic stimulation such as pain, anxiety, hypoxia, hypercarbia, hypoglycemia, or postictal state results in elevated blood pressure. Treating the underlying condition should resolve a pseudoemergency.

Special Situations

In cocaine-induced hypertensive emergencies, consider IV diltiazem, NTG, or nitroprusside. Avoid beta-blockers, which may result in unopposed alpha activity. Labetalol blocks both alpha and beta receptors and is acceptable.

In a pheochromocytoma crisis, give phentolamine 5–10 mg IV and repeat as needed. You can add sodium nitroprusside if needed. Avoid beta-blockers until after phentolamine is on board to prevent unopposed alpha activity.

Select labetalol or hydralazine IV for preeclampsia and eclampsia. Remember that ACE inhibitors and ARBs are contraindicated in pregnancy and should not be used.

Orthostatic Hypotension

One of the adverse effects associated with the management of hypertension is orthostatic hypotension. Orthostatic hypotension is an abnormal drop in BP that is symptomatic and occurs with standing. It is defined as a reduction of the systolic BP by 20 mmHg or more or a reduction of the diastolic BP by 10 mmHg or more when going from sitting to standing or lying to sitting. Diuretics and ACE inhibitors are commonly implicated.

Orthostatic hypotension is not always a result of antihypertensive medications. Psychotropic medications may cause orthostasis. Reduced blood volume, as in vomiting, diarrhea, or diaphoresis may result in orthostasis as well. If the drop in blood pressure is accompanied by an increase in the pulse rate of greater than 15 bpm, then it is likely due to depleted blood volume rather than as a result of medications.

Symptoms of orthostasis include dizziness, syncope, or the inability to stand for more than 1–2 minutes. Healthy subjects may not have symptoms unless the systolic BP drops below 70 mmHg.

Orthostatic hypotension can be diagnosed by obtaining orthostatic vital signs. If the diagnosis is not straightforward, a tilt table test may be helpful.

Management is directed at preventing syncope and treating the underlying problem. Adjustment of medications, increased fluid intake, support hose to avoid venous pooling, and fall precautions are often necessary. Fludrocortisone (Florinef) and octreotide may be used when necessary.

Chapter 18

Lipid Disorders

Introduction

Abnormal cholesterol levels, especially elevated low-density lipoprotein (LDL) levels and low high-density lipoprotein (HDL) levels, are associated with an increased risk of coronary heart disease, cerebrovascular disease, and peripheral vascular disease. Aggressive management of abnormal lipid levels by reducing total cholesterol and LDL cholesterol and by raising HDL cholesterol results in a reduction in myocardial infarction, angina, and stroke rates.

BACK TO THE BASICS

Lipids, such as cholesterol, also have an important role in the normal function of the human body. They are the building blocks of all fatty substances and are stored in the body to serve as sources of energy. They are essential in bile acid formation, which aids in the digestion of fats. Cholesterol is also essential for normal cell membrane function, steroid hormone production, and the formation of vitamin D. It may also be important for learning and memory.

Lipids are poorly soluble in the bloodstream so they require lipoproteins to transport them. Lipoproteins surround the lipids with a hydrophilic layer that is soluble in the bloodstream allowing for transport. There are five major lipoproteins, which are categorized by their size and density. The chylomicrons are the largest but least dense of the lipoproteins. The very low-density lipoproteins (VLDL) and intermediate density lipoproteins often transport triglycerides. LDL is the main transporter of cholesterol to the body and is often called the "bad" cholesterol while HDL is responsible for reverse

(continues)

> ## BACK TO THE BASICS (continued)
>
> cholesterol transport and is commonly referred to as the "good" cholesterol. Instead of delivering the cholesterol to the body, HDL scavenges excess cholesterol and transports it to the liver where it is excreted in the form of bile acids. HDL is the smallest but most dense of the lipoproteins.
>
> Lipoprotein (a) is essentially an LDL with a glycoprotein attached; it has a size and density between that of LDL and HDL. It carries apolipoprotein (a), which may interfere with the dissolution of blood clots.

Clinical Presentation

Although you may notice xanthomas on exam or observe the physical signs associated with the metabolic syndrome, most patients are asymptomatic and have no outward signs of a lipid disorder until vascular disease develops. For this reason, screening is essential.

Lipid Screening Guidelines

A fasting lipid profile should be obtained every 5 years for all people age 20 years and older. If the patient does not have coronary heart disease and their lipid levels are at goal, then recheck in 5 years. If their lipid levels are borderline or high and the patient has less than two risk factors, then recheck in 1 to 2 years. In high-risk patients or those with markedly elevated cholesterol, more frequent follow-up is recommended.

Diagnosis

If lipid levels are elevated, consider the possibility of an underlying cause. Medical conditions that may cause hypercholesterolemia include hypothyroidism, polycystic ovarian syndrome, obstructive liver disease, nephrotic disease, anorexia nervosa, or acute intermittent porphyria. Medications such as progestins, glucocorticoids, thiazide diuretics, or beta-blockers can also cause hypercholesterolemia.

Many people who develop coronary disease have cholesterol values that are at goal. For this reason, further testing may be required in patients who appear to be at goal, particularly if they have a family or personal history of heart disease.

Although it is not an independent risk factor, studies have shown that elevated LDL particle numbers and small, dense LDL size also predict coronary risk. Lipoprotein particle size and density may be obtained to determine if patients have the more atherogenic small, dense LDL despite having LDL levels that appear to be at goal. The NMR LipoProfile test screens for particle size and density.

Elevated levels of C-reactive protein (CRP), a nonspecific inflammatory marker, have been associated with a higher risk of MI, regardless of cholesterol levels. Elevated levels are associated with diabetes mellitus, central obesity, smoking, and estrogen.

Homocysteine may be toxic to the endothelium and levels can be lowered simply with folate and vitamin B_6 supplementation. However, lower levels of homocysteine may not translate into a reduction of CHD risk.

Increased levels of lipoprotein (a) have been associated with a higher risk of CHD and very high levels have been seen in families with a history of early onset vascular disease. Niacin lowers levels of lipoprotein (a), but a statin should be used initially because lowering the LDL level will reduce the risk of CHD in these patients. All first-degree relatives should be screened as well.

Treatment Goals

Although ideal total cholesterol is less than 200 mg/dL and levels above 240 mg/dL are considered high, it is essential to obtain a complete lipid panel to effectively diagnose and treat lipid disorders.

The primary goal of therapy is reduction of the LDL to target. Because the risk of CHD is increased when multiple risk factors are present, the treatment goal for LDL is based on the patient's number of cardiac risk factors; the higher their risk of CHD, the lower their LDL goal.

LDL treatment goals based on number of risk factors present:

0 to 1 risk factors	less than 160 mg/dL
2 or more risk factors	less than 130 mg/dL
Very high risk: Patients with known CHD or CHD risk equivalents	less than 100 mg/dL

CHD risk factors include cigarette smoking, hypertension, family history of premature CHD, age (men >45 years, women >55 years), and low HDL (<40).

CHD risk equivalents include noncoronary vascular disease such as symptomatic carotid artery disease (Stroke/TIA), abdominal aortic aneurysm, and peripheral vascular disease. Diabetes, metabolic syndrome, and chronic renal insufficiency (Cr >1.5) are also considered CHD risk equivalents.

Aggressive lipid-lowering therapy is required in patients who have known CHD or a CHD risk equivalent. The target LDL is less than 100 mg/dL and it has been proposed that patients with CHD who are at very high risk should achieve a goal of less than 70 mg/dL.

Triglyceride levels greater than 500 mg/dL should be aggressively treated to avoid the development of pancreatitis. Otherwise, it is preferable to focus on achieving the LDL goal before considering further treatment of triglycerides.

The following is the classification of triglyceride levels:

Normal	< 150 mg/dL
Borderline high	150 to 199 mg/dL
High	200 to 499 mg/dL
Very high	> 500 mg/dL

Low HDL levels are associated with increased risk of CHD. HDL goals are to achieve a level greater than 40 mg/dL in men and greater than 50 mg/dL in women. Elevated levels of HDL cholesterol actually lower the risk of CHD. In fact, a very high HDL (> 60 mg/dL) is considered a "negative" risk factor for CHD and one risk factor can be subtracted when calculating the LDL goal.

Management

Therapeutic Lifestyle Change

Therapeutic lifestyle changes are indicated in patients with abnormal lipoprotein levels and those with cardiac risk factors. Drug therapy should not be postponed if the target for LDL-C lowering is unlikely to be achieved soon with lifestyle changes alone. Crucial lifestyle changes include smoking cessation, diet, and exercise, which are discussed further in Chapter 27.

Medications

Rather than waiting for a trial of lifestyle changes, it is recommended that cholesterol-lowering medications be started along with a diet and exercise regimen in patients who are at higher risk. The guidelines suggest that the following scenarios warrant immediate medical therapy:

- LDL levels of 130 mg/dL or greater in patients with existing heart disease, diabetes, or another form of vascular disease (such as peripheral vascular disease or carotid artery disease).

- LDL levels of 160 mg/dL or greater in patients with two or more risk factors for heart disease.
- LDL levels of 190 mg/dL or greater in all patients.

Statins (HMG CoA Reductase Inhibitors)

Statins are the most commonly used drugs in the treatment of hypercholesterolemia. Statins are indicated for both primary and secondary prevention of CHD. They have been shown to reduce total mortality, MI, revascularization procedures, stroke, and peripheral vascular disease. They are the most powerful drugs for lowering LDL-C, with reductions of about 20–60%. Some statins are also able to raise the HDL by 5–15% and lower triglycerides by 7–30%.

Statins work by decreasing the body's synthesis of cholesterol and increasing the clearance of LDL from the bloodstream. They also reduce endothelial dysfunction, which is the first step in clot formation, and are effective at lowering CRP levels by reducing inflammation.

The following are all examples of statins: Lovastatin (Mevacor and Altoprev), pravastatin (Pravachol), simvastatin (Zocor), fluvastatin (Lescol), atorvastatin (Lipitor), and rosuvastatin (Crestor). Atorvastatin and rosuvastatin are the most potent statins currently on the market. Lovastatin and pravastatin are now available in generic form. The polypill Caduet consists of atorvastatin and amlodipine (Norvasc).

Statins are generally well tolerated and have fewer side effects than other cholesterol-lowering medications; however, myalgias and arthralgias are commonly encountered. *Myositis*, which is the term used for myalgias that are associated with a significantly elevated CK level, is rare but extremely important to identify because the statin must be discontinued to avoid progression to rhabdomyolysis. Rhabdomyolysis is myositis with an elevated creatinine level, which may lead to renal failure and death. The risk of myopathy is increased in patients who are frail, elderly, on multiple medications, have multisystem disease, or are undergoing major surgery.

Although rare, the risk of rhabdomyolysis increases substantially when statins are used in combination with certain medications. Many of these drug interactions involve the 3A4 isozyme of the cytochrome P450 system, which is responsible for the metabolism of many drugs in the liver. Simvastatin and lovastatin are both metabolized by this enzyme system and therefore the concentration of these drugs can increase dramatically in the presence of substances that inhibit CYP3A4. The following are examples of medications that should be used with caution in patients on simvastatin and lovastatin: itraconazole (Sporanox) and ketaconazole (Nizoral), macrolide antibiotics, erythromycin and clarithromycin (Biaxin), HIV protease inhibitors, verapamil, amiodarone, and nefazodone

(Serzone). Grapefruit juice is also metabolized through the cytochrome P450 system and therefore large quantities should be avoided. The other statins are metabolized partially or completely by alternate pathways and are less affected by other medications. Gemfibrozil (Lopid) and cyclosporine (i.e., Sandimmune) raise the risk of rhabdomyolysis in all statins.

GI complaints, fatigue, headache, and rash may also occur. Although rare, polyneuropathy, memory loss, sleep disturbances, impotence, gynecomastia, lupus-like syndrome, and pancreatitis have been reported.

Pearl

When initiating statin therapy, warn patients to notify you immediately if they develop new or worsening myalgias. If these symptoms arise, order a CK level and hold the statin until you can confirm it is safe to resume. Also consider checking a TSH level because hypothyroidism may predispose patients to myopathy.

Absolute contraindications are active or chronic liver disease. Relative contraindications include the concomitant use of cyclosporine, gemfibrozil, niacin, macrolide antibiotics, many antifungal agents, and other cytochrome P450 inhibitors. Most statins should be used in lower doses for those patients with severe kidney disease.

Pearl

Check the package insert periodically on the statin that you are prescribing; drug interactions and black-box warnings are frequently updated.

Bile Acid Sequestrants

The bile acid sequestrants are commonly called *resins*. They bind and eliminate bile acids in the intestine; the absence of bile acids mobilizes the cholesterol in the bloodstream to form bile, thus eliminating the cholesterol from the body.

Resins can lower the LDL by up to 20% and increase HDL levels, but may worsen triglyceride levels in patients with hypertriglyceridemia. Cholestyramine (Prevalite, Questran, Questran Light), colestipol (Colestid), and colesevelam (Welchol) are all examples of resins.

Use is often limited by GI side effects which include nausea, bloating, cramping, eructations, constipation, and heartburn. Colesevelam is a newer agent that is better tolerated than the others. Increasing fluid intake and adding stool softeners often aids in patient tolerance but drug discontinuation is common.

Bottom Line

Order a lipid panel and a liver panel prior to initiation of therapy. Monitor the AST/ALT at 3 months and then annually or, if indicated, clinically. If elevated liver enzymes are noted, reduce the dose or try a different agent with careful attention to liver enzymes during follow-up. The statin dose should be titrated every 4 to 6 weeks to achieve the goal.

Cholestyramine and colestipol decrease the absorption of other medications; therefore, take other medications 1–2 hours before or 4–6 hours after taking cholestyramine or colestipol. Malabsorption of fat-soluble vitamins may occur with high doses. Plasma folate levels are decreased with resins and supplementation should be considered, particularly in children and women of childbearing age.

Bottom Line

Bile acid sequestrants should be avoided in hypertriglyceridemia. Patient tolerance is a major factor limiting the use of resins, but Colesevelam is better tolerated than other resins. Consider folate supplementation with the use of resins.

Nicotinic Acid (Niacin)

Niacin reduces the metabolism of VLDL in the liver, which reduces the amount of LDL that is synthesized. It also interferes with the breakdown of HDL. Although it lowers VLDL and LDL, it is predominantly used to raise HDL. Low HDL is an independent risk factor for CHD and is a secondary goal in managing dyslipidemia.

Flushing and GI complaints are common with niacin. Pruritis, blurred vision, fatigue, glucose intolerance, hyperuricemia, hepatic toxicity, and exacerbation of peptic ulcers may also occur. Niaspan is an extended release formulation that has significantly less flushing or hepatotoxicity in doses less than 2 grams per day. Advicor is a polypill consisting of lovastatin and extended release niacin.

Regular monitoring of liver function is required with niacin and it is contraindicated in patients with active liver disease. Exercise caution in patients with diabetes, because it may worsen glycemic control by causing

Pearl

To diminish flushing, take aspirin about 30 minutes prior to niacin and take niacin after meals.

insulin resistance. Niacin may precipitate active arthritis in people with gout, may exacerbate angina, and may cause hypotension if taken concomitantly with vasodilators.

Fibrates

Fibrates regulate the genes that are responsible for lipid metabolism. They lower triglyceride levels, raise HDL levels, and shift the LDL toward a less atherogenic type. Fibrates are used primarily for severe hypertriglyceridemia, especially when concern for the development of pancreatitis exists. Smaller elevations of triglycerides are typically managed with statins. Fibrates are also used to raise HDL levels.

Gemfibrozil (Lopid) and fenofibrate (TriCor) are both fibrates. Adverse effects, which include GI disturbances, cholelithiasis, hepatitis, and myositis, are more common with gemfibrozil than fenofibrate.

Lower doses should be used in patients who are taking oral hypoglycemics or anticoagulants or in those patients with renal disease.

Gemfibrozil inhibits the metabolism of statins in the liver, but fenofibrate does not. Therefore, if concomitant use of a statin and a fibrate is necessary, choose fenofibrate to reduce the risk of myositis and rhabdomyolysis.

Cholesterol Absorption Inhibitor

Ezitimibe (Zetia) inhibits intestinal absorption of cholesterol. It is currently the only agent in this class other than Vytorin, the polypill that contains ezetimibi with simvastatin. It is primarily used to lower LDL in conjunction with a statin or when a statin is not tolerated. Ezetimibi lowers LDL (18%), but has limited benefit on triglycerides or HDL.

Flatulence is the most common adverse reaction, otherwise, it is typically well tolerated. There have been reports of myalgias, rhabdomyolysis, hepatitis, pancreatitis, and thrombocytopenia. Avoid use in moderate to severe liver dysfunction. Cyclosporine increases blood levels. Absorption is decreased if bile acid sequestrants are taken within a few hours. Myalgias may occur if used concomitantly with statins.

Omega-3 Fatty Acids

Omega-3 fatty acids have been shown to reduce cholesterol, triglycerides, and LDL levels and may even raise HDL. Omega-3 fatty acids are present in dietary fish oil, OTC supplements, and prescription Omacor. Dietary fish consumption has also been shown to reduce the risk of CHD. Excessive doses (15–30 g/day) have caused thrombocytopenia and bleeding disorders.

Fiber

Fiber absorbs water in the colon leading to bulkier stools. It lowers LDL cholesterol levels by binding bile acids and reducing cholesterol absorption. Fiber also slows the rate of carbohydrate absorption, which helps prevent insulin surges. Fiber has the added benefit of increasing satiety without contributing calories.

Red Yeast Rice

Red yeast rice (monascus purpureus) contains the same chemical as the drug lovastatin (Mevacor). Studies have shown that red yeast rice lowers LDL and total cholesterol levels. Adverse reactions may be similar to those of lovastatin and red yeast may also increase the risk of bleeding.

Miscellaneous Agents to Reduce Cholesterol

Artichoke extract, barley, garlic extract, and oat bran may all reduce the total cholesterol as well as LDL levels.

Lipid Lowering with Comorbidities

Statins are generally prescribed for all CHD patients regardless of the LDL cholesterol level. In the setting of an acute MI, begin high-dose statin immediately, regardless of cholesterol level.

Diabetes mellitus is considered a CHD "equivalent"; therefore, people with diabetes mellitus are treated as if they have CHD.

A patient with a limited life span from a concomitant illness is probably not a candidate for drug therapy. On the other hand, an otherwise healthy, elderly individual should not be denied drug therapy on the basis of age alone.

Chapter 19

Atherosclerosis and Coronary Heart Disease

Introduction

A student once mentioned that learning cardiology was like learning a foreign language. She felt that the subject matter would be much simpler to grasp if she had a working knowledge of the "lingo" before delving into more difficult concepts. Consequently, this section begins with a little bit of "lingo" as the groundwork for learning more advanced cardiac concepts.

BACK TO THE BASICS

Atherosclerosis

Atherosclerosis is the narrowing and blockage of arteries by plaque, which consists of cholesterol, calcium, clotting proteins, and other substances. These deposits build up on the inner lining of the artery, the endothelium, beginning in childhood and progressing throughout life.

The process of atherosclerosis begins with the development of fatty streaks, which are thin, flat, yellow discolorations on the inner lining of the artery. The fatty streak then progresses to form a fibrous plaque, which is the basic lesion of atherosclerosis.

(continues)

BACK TO THE BASICS (continued)

As the plaque matures, it develops a lipid core and a fibrous cap. Eventually, it may grow large enough to begin encroaching upon the lumen of the artery resulting in impeded blood flow. Atherosclerosis is generally asymptomatic until the plaque stenosis exceeds 70–80%. Lesions of this size, if present in a coronary artery, can produce ischemia.

Ischemia

A blood vessel that is occluded by atherosclerosis may cause a temporary lack of blood flow to areas of the heart that are supplied by the vessel. The temporary lack of blood flow may cause ischemia if oxygen demand exceeds this limited supply. Ischemia often causes chest pain that is described as angina.

Ischemic chest pain will resolve as soon as blood flow is restored to the area. Blood flow may be restored either by reducing oxygen demand (i.e., resting) or by increasing oxygen supply (i.e., taking nitroglycerine, which dilates the coronary arteries allowing more room for blood to pass through). Ischemia is typically short-lived without sufficient time for cell death to occur. If blood flow is not restored, then cell death (infarction) may occur.

Bottom Line

Atherosclerosis is the "junk that accumulates in an artery" and CHD is the disease that occurs when this "junk" deposits in a coronary artery. CHD is sometimes also referred to as coronary artery disease (CAD). Angina is a description of the pain that accompanies CHD.

Angina

Angina is the term for the classic symptoms of chest pain that occur with coronary ischemia. These symptoms are described in Chapter 12.

Coronary Heart Disease

Coronary heart disease (CHD), sometimes called *coronary artery disease,* is a term that encompasses both stable angina pectoris and acute coronary syndrome, which includes ST-elevation MI, non-ST elevation myocardial infarction, and unstable angina. It is the leading cause of death in the United States.

Stable Angina

Stable angina is a clinical syndrome that arises when a fixed plaque occludes a portion of a coronary artery resulting in the inability to meet oxygen demand during exertion. At rest, less oxygen is required to meet the heart's needs, so the blockage does not result in clinical symptoms. However, with the increased oxygen demands that exertion imposes, there is just not enough room to squeeze more blood past the blockage (stenosis). This lack of oxygen causes ischemia in the areas of the heart that are supplied by the occluded coronary artery.

Acute Coronary Syndrome

When the endothelium of an artery becomes injured, an inflammatory cascade ensues. This may cause the fibrous cap of the plaque to rupture, allowing the lipid core to spill out, which is called *thrombosis*. Platelets aggregate at the area of thrombosis, leading to clot formation, thus, compromising blood flow. The lack of blood flow that results from this process of thrombosis and clot formation causes a clinical syndrome known as *acute coronary syndrome (ACS)*. ACS is a continuum of disease ranging from unstable angina (UA) to myocardial infarction (MI).

Unstable Angina

Unstable angina is considered to be present in patients with ischemic symptoms suggestive of ACS, but without ST elevation or elevation of cardiac enzymes (troponin or CK-MB).

> **Pearl**
> Stable angina results from a supply-demand mismatch; it is exertional, exertional, exertional!

> **Bottom Line**
> If a patient develops new symptoms that occur at rest or markedly limit physical activity or if a patient presents with worsening symptoms of previously stable angina, then you may be dealing with ACS, which is an unstable, potentially life-threatening condition requiring admission.

Non-ST Elevation MI

Non-ST Elevation MI (NSTEMI) is considered to be present in patients with ischemic symptoms suggestive of ACS and an elevation in cardiac enzymes, but without ST elevation on EKG.

UA and NSTEMI differ primarily in whether the ischemia is severe enough to cause sufficient myocardial damage to release detectable quantities of cardiac enzymes (troponin or CK-MB).

ST Elevation MI

In ST segment elevation MI (STEMI), plaque rupture results in complete occlusion and obstruction of the vessel. This results in death (necrosis) of the area of myocardium that was supplied by the occluded vessel due to a complete loss of the supply of oxygen from that vessel.

(continues)

BACK TO THE BASICS (continued)

Infarct

An infarct occurs when an occlusion causes lack of blood flow that lasts long enough to cause the heart cells to die. NSTEMI and STEMI are examples of myocardial infarctions.

Vasospastic Coronary Disease

Vasospastic coronary disease (Prinzmetal's angina or variant angina) occurs when a coronary artery has a spasm, which causes temporary occlusion and loss of blood supply to the myocardium that is supplied by that blood vessel. Vasospasm is a less common cause of angina.

Bottom Line

Stable angina	Supply-demand mismatch, but no thrombosis or clotting has occurred	Exertional symptoms	No ST elevation	Normal cardiac enzymes
Unstable angina*	Thrombosis/clot has occurred	Unstable symptoms	No ST elevation	Normal cardiac enzymes
NSTEMI*	Thrombosis/clot has occurred	Unstable symptoms	No ST elevation	Abnormal cardiac enzymes
STEMI*	Thrombosis/clot has occurred	Persistent symptoms	ST elevation	Abnormal cardiac enzymes

*Part of the continuum of acute coronary syndrome

Clinical Manifestations of Atherosclerosis

Atherosclerosis of coronary arteries, CHD, may present as stable angina, ACS, or in the worst-case scenario, sudden death. Stable angina typically presents as exertional chest pain or dyspnea. The presentation of classic angina is described in Chapter 12. ACS is recognizable clinically by the new onset of angina symptoms that markedly limit physical activity or the escalation of previous angina symptoms. In a patient with previously stable angina, ACS becomes a concern when the stable pattern becomes unstable as manifested by increasing severity or frequency of angina episodes, less exertion provoking episodes, or by symptoms occurring at rest or awakening the patient from sleep.

Atherosclerosis may also affect other blood vessels. Cerebrovascular disease may present with a cerebrovascular accident (stroke) or transient ischemic attack (TIA). Peripheral vascular disease may present as intermittent claudication or pain in the calves when walking that is relieved within a few minutes of rest.

Pearl

If the history, physical, and EKG suggest that the patient is experiencing ACS, activate EMS (call 911) and begin treatment while awaiting their arrival. "Time is muscle"; you must supply blood to the myocardium as soon as possible to avoid necrosis of the muscle.

Diagnosis and Management Strategy

In order to formulate a diagnostic and treatment plan, the type of CHD must first be identified.

Stable angina is easily distinguished from ACS by symptoms. Because the clinical presentation is the same in unstable angina, NSTEMI, and STEMI, an EKG and serial cardiac enzymes are essential to differentiate between them. The EKG will immediately differentiate STEMI from UA and NSTEMI. Cardiac enzymes are essential in differentiating between UA and NSTEMI because neither of these conditions causes elevation of the ST segments.

Cardiac enzymes may take up to 24 hours to elevate and treatment needs to begin immediately, so these two conditions are lumped together for management purposes.

Stable Angina
Initial Presentation

Aside from the initial EKG, stress testing with or without additional imaging is usually the first diagnostic study performed to assess patients with chest pain that is possibly ischemic. While waiting for diagnostic testing to be completed, patients with a clinical picture suggestive of stable angina should be placed on an aspirin (ASA), a beta-blocker, and NTG sublingual, unless contraindicated.

If an ischemic etiology is discovered during stress testing and revascularization is a consideration (either with percutaneous intervention or bypass surgery), then cardiac catheterization may be considered.

> **Pearl**
>
> Occasionally, the clinical presentation warrants proceeding directly to cardiac catheterization without performing a stress test. As you gain experience, you will become more comfortable making these decisions, but remember to corroborate with the cardiologist.

The following conditions may provoke or exacerbate angina and should be excluded during the initial presentation of angina: profound anemia, poorly controlled hypertension, hyperthyroidism, hypoxemia, arrhythmias, valvular heart disease, and hypertrophic cardiomyopathy. Excessive thyroid replacement, vasodilators, and vasoconstrictors may also result in angina.

If the diagnostic evaluation confirms that the patient's chest pain is indeed due to angina, the following medications are recommended:

- Aspirin: reduces the risk of cardiovascular events and stroke; no antiplatelet therapy has been proven superior to aspirin
- Clopidogrel (Plavix): can be substituted if the patient has a true aspirin allergy
- Beta-blocker: for control of ischemic pain and reduction of morbidity and mortality, particularly if they have had a prior MI
- ACE inhibitor: in patients with concomitant diabetes or systolic dysfunction; also in patients with a history of an MI, to reduce the likelihood of recurrent MI, cardiac arrest, and death
- Angiotensin receptor blocker: in patients who have had an MI and have heart failure or systolic dysfunction if they are unable to tolerate an ACE inhibitor
- Statin: to achieve their target cholesterol goals
- Sublingual nitroglycerine: to take as needed for angina
- Long-acting nitrate: may be added to reduce myocardial oxygen demand if additional symptom relief is required or if the patient is unable to take a beta-blocker
- Dihydropyridine CCB: may be added if additional symptom relief is required, but it does not improve survival

> **Pearl**
> When treating vasospastic CHD, choose a CCB rather than a beta-blocker.

For Example

Antiplatelets: aspirin 75 to 162 mg po daily or clopidogrel (Plavix) 75 mg orally daily

Beta-blockers: metoprolol 50 mg po BID or Toprol XL 50 mg po QD

ACE inhibitor: lisinopril 2.5 or 5 mg po QD

Nitrates: Imdur 60 mg po qd or isosorbide dinitrate 20 mg po BID take first dose in morning and last dose at dinnertime

CCBs: Norvasc (amlodipine) 5 mg po qd

Pearl

Always avoid short-acting CCBs, because they have had negative outcomes.

Pearl

Prescribe NTG sublingual and instruct the patient to use it if they have an episode of chest pain that does not resolve with rest within several minutes. Inform them to activate EMS if symptoms are not improved after 1 tablet. They may then repeat the NTG two times every 5 minutes until the chest pain is resolved.

Follow-Up Visit

The following should be accomplished during a follow-up visit for stable CHD:

- Determine whether the patient is having any cardiac or vascular symptoms.
- Assess functional class.
- Review medications.
- Address psychosocial issues.
- Discuss physical limitations.
- Employ secondary prevention strategies including cardiac risk factor modification, lifestyle changes, and cardiac rehabilitation.
- Assess the patient's risk for future cardiac events.
- Make sure patients and family are aware of ischemic symptoms to monitor and have a cardiac emergency response plan.

Symptoms

Patients with CHD are at high risk for developing future cardiovascular events as well as other vascular diseases. Ask specifically if the patient has been having any exertional symptoms, CP, dyspnea, orthopnea, PND, edema, intermittent claudication, dizziness, syncope, palpitations, fatigue, or weakness.

If the patient is having chest pain, consider asking some of the following questions to determine whether the symptoms are progressing and warrant further evaluation:

- Is the pain the same as when you had your heart problem in the past?
- How often are you taking your NTG? Is this more than last time you were seen?
- Has the pattern of your chest pain changed since you had your stent or angioplasty?
- What is the most active thing that you do in a day and does this activity result in symptoms?

Functional Classification

Determine the patient's functional status using the New York Heart Association Classification scheme. Patients are classified as class I if they have no limitation of activity; class II means a slight limitation of physical activity (i.e., climbing stairs); class III is marked limitation of activity (i.e., walking across a room); and Class IV is reserved for patients with symptoms at rest.

Medications

Review the patient's medication list to ensure that the patient is on all medications that have a proven benefit in improving morbidity and/or mortality and titrate them as needed. Ensure the patient is able to afford medications, understands their importance, and is adherent to the medical regimen.

Pearl

Although it is easy for patients to see the benefits of drugs in acute care (i.e., sublingual NTG for chest pain), the benefits are not visible with chronic, preventative care. Cardiac patients are often on a cocktail of drugs for secondary prevention and need constant reminders of their benefits to avoid the inclination to discontinue them.

Pearl

Hormone therapy was once felt to confer protection against coronary artery disease and was actually prescribed for that purpose. It is now known that the opposite is true; therefore, estrogen plus progestin should not be given to postmenopausal women for secondary prevention of coronary events. Additionally, if a postmenopausal woman is admitted with an MI, discontinue her estrogen plus progestin hormone therapy if applicable.

Pearl

Regular use of ibuprofen should be avoided because it blocks the antiplatelet effects of aspirin. (Intermittent use is OK.)

Psychosocial Status

Patients with CHD should be routinely assessed for concomitant depression, anxiety, or sleep disorders. Ensure that the patient has a social support system in place. Cardiac rehab programs are an excellent way for patients to connect with other people who have had similar medical problems.

Physical Limitations

Patients with CHD are frequently concerned about physical limitations, their ability to return to work, the safety of sexual activity, and traveling. Use an individualized approach based on functional status, comorbidities, and type of employment in order to address these concerns.

In patients with a recent MI, daily walking can be encouraged immediately after discharge. However, heavy lifting or bending should be avoided for 48 hours after catheterization. Exercise should be limited by the development of symptoms. If these restrictions do not hamper employment, and the patient is asymptomatic while working, then the patient may be able to safely return to work.

Consider performing an exercise treadmill test to assess a patient's exercise tolerance prior to enrolling in cardiac rehab or initiating a home exercise program.

It is generally believed that if a patient can walk up several flights of stairs without symptoms that they are able to engage in sexual activity. Advise patients that if they are taking a phosphodiesterase inhibitor for sexual function and develop angina, they will not be able to safely take nitroglycerine.

Patients should not drive for 48 hours after catheterization and should avoid prolonged sitting, which often accompanies travel, for 1 week.

Secondary Prevention

Smoking cessation, aggressive lipid lowering, and control of hypertension and diabetes have proven beneficial in secondary prevention of CHD. Additionally, benefit has been shown with prophylactic use of aspirin, beta-blockers, ACE inhibitors, and statins.

Lifestyle modifications including diet, exercise, smoking cessation, stress reduction, and weight management promote a less atherogenic and less pro-thrombotic state. Weight reduction enhances lowering of other risk factors for cardiovascular disease, including LDL-C, triglycerides, glucose, and blood pressure.

Encourage a diet that is low in saturated fat and cholesterol along with increased consumption of omega-3 fatty acids, fruits, vegetables, soluble (viscous) fiber, and whole grains. Patients should strive to balance calorie intake with energy output in order to achieve and maintain a healthy weight.

All-cause mortality is reduced up to 40% by an increase in weekly energy expenditure from 500 kcal to 2000 kcal. Cardiac rehabilitation is an excellent means of starting or resuming an exercise program in patients who have had an MI or an intervention. For additional guidance on lifestyle changes, see Chapter 27.

A lipid profile should be performed or obtained from recent past records. Management of lipids is discussed in Chapter 18.

All patients with CHD should be advised to stop smoking and to avoid secondhand smoke. Smoking triggers coronary spasm and doubles mortality rates after an MI. Smoking also reduces the anti-ischemic effects of beta-blockers.

Blood pressure should be treated with drug therapy to less than 140/90 mmHg and to less than 130/80 mmHg for patients with diabetes or chronic kidney disease. Lifestyle modification should be initiated in all patients with blood pressure greater than or equal to 120/80 mmHg.

Tight glucose control in diabetics during and after an MI has been shown to lower acute and 1-year mortality rates and reduces microvascular disease. The goal of diabetes management is to achieve a HbA1C less than 7%.

Risk Assessment

Within 6 years of sustaining a heart attack, 18% of men and 35% of women will have another heart attack and 6–7% will experience sudden death. The survival rate for sudden cardiac arrest that occurs outside of the hospital is very low (5%). This is because, in order to have hope for resuscitation, defibrillation needs to occur within 6–8 minutes.

Functional classification and left ventricular function can be used to assess a patient's risk for sudden cardiac death. NYHA class I patients have a 20% mortality rate at 5 years while 40–50% of patients with class IV symptoms will not survive another year. Patients with a reduced left ventricular EF are also at high risk for sudden cardiac death.

Patients with an EF less than 35% and class II to III heart failure who are already optimized on medications are at high risk of mortality. These high-risk patients should be considered for an implantable cardioverter-defibrillator (ICD), which has been shown to be 99% effective in preventing sudden cardiac death.

Emergency Response Plan

Be sure patients and their loved ones or caregivers are able to identify acute ischemic symptoms and know the appropriate steps to take should these symptoms occur. They should know how and when to activate EMS (i.e., if chest pain is not relieved by three NTG administered sublingually 5 minutes apart).

Patients should carry a card in their wallets identifying stents, pacemakers, valves, ICDs, or other devices. Additionally, they should have a list of their past medical history, medications, allergies, family member's contact information, and physicians' contact information visible on the refrigerator and in their wallets. If patients have an abnormal baseline EKG, it is wise to carry a shrunken laminated copy in their wallets.

Family members of patients with a history of an MI should be advised to obtain CPR or automated external defibrillator (AED) training and should be given community resources to obtain this training.

Pearl

Remember **ABCDE** when managing stable angina:

A: **A**spirin, **A**CE inhibitor, and **A**ntianginal

B: **B**eta-blocker and **B**P control

C: **C**holesterol agent and **C**igarette cessation

D: **D**iabetes and **D**iet management

E: **E**xercise and **E**ducation

Unstable Angina and Non-ST Elevation MI

Preliminary Management

A patient with UA/NSTEMI should be treated rapidly. Management goals include immediate relief of chest pain and prevention of recurrent ischemia and death. The cornerstones of therapy, therefore, include anti-ischemic and antithrombotic agents. The following basic steps should be undertaken immediately, prior to confirming the diagnosis:

- Assess ABCs (airway, breathing, and circulation).
- Obtain and interpret an EKG.

- Summon EMS and/or have a crash cart available.
- Administer oxygen (2 or 3 liters via nasal cannula is usually sufficient).
- Place the patient on a heart monitor.
- Obtain IV access.
- Draw blood for labwork if the patient is in the ED or an inpatient setting.
- Administer aspirin 162 mg–325 mg to chew and swallow.
- Administer sublingual nitroglycerin 0.4 mg every 5 minutes for a total of three doses, and then decide whether to add intravenous nitroglycerin or nitropaste. (Your decision will be based on whether the patient's blood pressure will allow more nitrates, whether symptoms are still present, and how likely the patient is having an MI.)
- Continually monitor the patient's vital signs and symptoms. Ask the patient to rate pain on a scale of 1 to 10 and document the pain level and vital signs periodically and after each therapeutic agent is given.
- Add an IV beta-blocker followed by an oral beta-blocker (i.e., metoprolol 5 mg IV followed by 25 mg po QD) if the patient's pulse and blood pressure will allow it.
- Provide morphine sulfate (i.e., 2–4 mg IV stat and repeat every 2–4 hours as needed) to relieve agitation or manage pain that is not immediately relieved by nitroglycerine and beta-blockers.

Initial History And Exam

A cursory history and physical exam should be performed to confirm the initial assessment, determine any past history of cardiovascular disease or risk factors for cardiovascular disease, and to assess for potential contraindications to thrombolytic therapy if it is being considered. Determine the attributes of the pain including associated symptoms and continually assess the severity of pain as treatment is provided.

Physical examination should include an assessment of the patient's hemodynamic status, a cardiovascular exam, pulmonary auscultation, and a screening neurologic examination.

Diagnostic Studies

Labwork should include cardiac enzymes, PT/INR/PTT, electrolytes including magnesium, BUN/Cr, and a lipid panel.

The most commonly used cardiac enzymes are troponin and CK-MB. Cardiac enzymes must be evaluated serially over a 24-hour period because they do not elevate right away. Order the enzymes at baseline and every 6–8 hours within a 24-hour period.

The EKG may reveal ST depression or t-wave inversion in patients with angina or non-ST elevation MI. ST segment elevation will be evident in an ST elevation infarction. Q waves may indicate an old MI or an evolving new MI.

Differential Diagnosis of Angina

Cocaine and amphetamine use may increase myocardial oxygen demand or cause vasospasm leading to angina. Acute pulmonary disorders or carbon monoxide poisoning may result in hypoxia, which can cause angina. Ventricular hypertrophy due to cardiomyopathy, hypertension, or valvular heart disease may also cause angina. Severe anemia may cause angina if underlying coronary disease is present.

Definitive Management

Once a diagnosis of UA or NSTEMI is confirmed by elevation of the cardiac enzymes, a few medications will need to be added to the preliminary regimen. These include heparin or low-molecular weight heparin (enoxaparin [Lovenox]), clopidogrel (Plavix), and possibly a glycoprotein IIb/IIIa inhibitor. A statin or other lipid-lowering agent may also be required.

When dealing with a higher-risk patient, cardiac catheterization with anticipated revascularization is preferable to noninvasive management. Higher-risk patients include those with recurrent angina, rest angina despite medical management, recurrent angina accompanied by congestive heart failure, new or worsening mitral regurgitation, an abnormal stress test, an EF less than 40%, hemodynamic instability, sustained ventricular tachycardia, ST depression on EKG, elevated troponin, percutaneous intervention in the past 6 months, or previous coronary artery bypass grafting surgery.

Pearl

I always write the following recommendation when I am asked to consult on a patient with anemia and underlying coronary disease: "Recommend keeping the hemoglobin greater than or equal to 10 from a cardiac standpoint."

Bottom Line

ACS/Unstable Angina Management

- Antiplatelet agents (ASA, plavix, glycoprotein 3b-2a inhibitors)
- Anticoagulant (Lovenox or heparin)
- Nitroglycerine
- Beta-blocker
- ACE inhibitor
- Statin or other lipid-lowering agent if applicable
- Referral for possible revascularization

Acute ST Elevation Myocardial Infarction

Once ST elevation is noted on the EKG, rapid management is essential. In acute STEMI, reperfusion therapy should not await the results of cardiac enzymes. Rapid reperfusion, complete and immediate relief of ischemic pain, and the correction of any hemodynamic abnormalities are all management priorities. Also, ensure electrolytes, particularly potassium and magnesium, are not low because this contributes to the development of life-threatening ventricular arrhythmias.

STEMI patients will need to be started rapidly on the following medications:

- Aspirin
- Clopidogrel (Plavix)
- Nitrates; for persistent pain, congestive heart failure, or hypertension, intravenous nitroglycerin can be given, provided there are no contraindications (use of drugs for erectile dysfunction or right ventricular infarction.) Start at 5 ml/hr and titrate to relief of pain keeping SBP >100. Discontinue the infusion if the patient becomes hypotensive.
- ACE inhibitor
- Beta-blocker; it is preferable to give a cardioselective intravenous beta-blocker initially (i.e., IV metoprolol 5 mg q 5mins x 3 or IV Atenolol 5mg). You may repeat either of these medications in 5 minutes and then follow each of these with oral beta-blockers.
- Heparin/ enoxaparin; heparin and aspirin interfere with thrombus formation at different sites and therefore are both used in the treatment of ACS.
- Morphine sulfate; morphine is added to ensure complete relief of chest pain. Give 2 to 5 mg IV every 5 to 30 minutes as needed.
- Glycoprotein IIb/IIIa inhibitors block the final common pathway in platelet aggregation. They have been shown to improve outcomes only when used in conjunction with other antiplatelets and are indicated in UA if there is >2mm ST depression on the EKG or in ST elevation MI awaiting PCI. These agents block further platelet aggregation, but do not dissolve existing clots. Therefore, a thrombolytic or PCI is still essential for reperfusion. Abcixamab (Reopro), eptifibatide (Integrilin), and tirofibran (Aggrastat) are all examples of GP IIb/IIIa inhibitors. Each of these agents has different indications so discuss which agent to use with your supervising physician or familiarize yourself with the package insert.
- High-dose statin

Unless contraindicated, start the patient on these medications immediately while deciding how to reperfuse the patient. This may be accomplished by either rushing the patient to the catheterization lab for primary percutaneous coronary intervention (PCI) or by administering thrombolytics.

Reperfusion Therapy

Time is a critical factor in managing STEMI patients. Benefit is significantly greater when reperfusion occurs within 4 hours of the onset of symptoms. All patients with an acute STEMI should undergo some sort of reperfusion therapy (PCI or thrombolysis) if less than 12 hours has elapsed from the onset of symptoms.

If your facility has immediate access to a catheterization lab, call the interventional cardiologist on call or the catheterization team to determine how long it will take to get the patient treated. If they will be unable to perform PCI within 90 minutes of initial contact or PCI will take more than an hour longer than it will take to give a thrombolytic, then a thrombolytic agent is preferred, unless contraindicated.

Contraindications to Thrombolytic Therapy

Absolute contraindications include the following:

- Active bleeding
- Defective hemostasis
- Recent major trauma
- Surgical or invasive procedure < 10 days ago
- Neurosurgical procedure < 2 months ago
- GI/GU bleeding within 6 months
- Prolonged CPR (> 10 minutes)
- TIA/CVA < 12 months ago
- Past history of a CNS tumor, aneurysm, or AVM
- Acute pericarditis
- Suspected aortic dissection
- Active peptic ulcer disease
- Active inflammatory bowel disease
- Active cavitary lung disease
- Pregnancy

Pearl

Most EDs have a checklist that you can grab in order to determine whether the patient is a candidate for antithrombotic therapy.

Pearl

Stress testing is used to diagnose stable angina or chest pain syndromes, but is contraindicated in acute MI.

Relative contraindications include the following:

- Systolic BP > 180 mmHg or diastolic BP > 110 mmHg
- Bacterial endocarditis
- Hemorrhagic diabetic retinopathy
- History of intraocular bleeding
- CVA/TIA > 12 months ago
- Brief CPR (< 10 minutes)
- Chronic coumadin use
- Severe renal or liver disease
- Severe menses

Cardiac Catheterization

Cardiac catheterization is performed with the intent to follow immediately with a percutaneous coronary intervention such as a stent or angioplasty.

Prognosis

Bradycardia or tachycardia, especially sustained ventricular tachycardia, hypotension, or signs of heart failure (new or worsening rales, MR murmur, S3 gallop) are all associated with an increased risk of death or reinfarction within 30 days of an MI.

Bottom Line

Acute MI

- Oxygen
- ASA
- Plavix (if not likely to need urgent CABG)
- Heparin or lovenox (Choose heparin if using a thrombotic)
- NTG
- Beta-blocker
- Morphine sulfate
- Thrombolytic or PCI
- ACE inhibitor
- Statin

Cardio Reality

As I walk into the exam room, I hear a squeal and look down at the little girl nestled in her carrier. She is a beautiful 3-month-old girl named Lila. Also in the exam room are Lila's father, who is seated next to her and her mother, who is seated on the exam table. Lila's mother is a 37-year-old who is here for follow-up of an acute MI that she sustained several weeks ago. Lila's mother also happens to be an ICU nurse. She was at work in the ICU when she developed severe chest pain. She walked over to the ED and immediately was taken back for evaluation. Her presentation was consistent with ACS but her symptoms did not improve with appropriate medical care. The decision was made to proceed with emergency cardiac catheterization, which revealed dissection of the right coronary artery from top to bottom. Four stents were utilized to reconstruct the artery and several postoperative complications ensued. Eventually, Lila's mother returned home to her husband and two young children.

If you are like me, you will find this story shocking. How can such a young woman have sustained such a horrifying cardiac event? Surely she must have a history of hypertension, right? Wrong. Then she must have been a smoker, right? Wrong again. Well, then she must have had a horrible family history of heart disease, right? Wrong again.

It turns out that spontaneous coronary artery dissection, although rare, occurs in relatively young people and has a predilection for women. Additionally, 31% of cases that occurred in women were associated with the postpartum state, but nobody knows why. It is known that hormonal changes during pregnancy cause microstructural changes in the aorta; it is possible that changes also occur in the coronary arteries and predispose women to dissection during the postpartum period.

So the next time you see a young person having an MI, particularly young women in the postpartum state, consider spontaneous coronary artery dissection in the differential diagnosis.

Chapter 20

Congestive Heart Failure

Introduction

Heart failure is a disabling and often deadly health care problem. Although the incidence of other cardiac illnesses is declining, heart failure incidence continues to rise. Heart failure afflicts more than 5 million Americans and is the leading reason for hospitalization of Americans over the age of 65.

The prognosis for patients with heart failure is poor. Because two thirds of patients are managed exclusively by primary care providers, it is clearly an illness that all PAs and NPs should be prepared to manage, regardless of specialization.

BACK TO THE BASICS

Causes of Heart Failure

Heart failure occurs when the heart is unable to pump enough blood to meet the oxygen demands of the body. This may be due to a problem with the ventricle obtaining enough blood to pump (diastolic failure) or a problem with the ventricle ejecting the blood (systolic failure). An increased workload or a myocardial disorder may lead to systolic failure while restriction of ventricular filling may lead to diastolic failure.

Increased workload may be due to hyperthyroidism, anemia, arteriovenous fistulas, valvular regurgitation, a left-to-right shunt, systemic or pulmonary hypertension, pulmonic or aortic stenosis, systemic infection, psychological stress, exercise (especially on hot, humid days), or a pulmonary embolism.

Myocardial insults that may lead to heart failure include myocardial infarction or ischemia, arrhythmias, hypoxia, infectious diseases such as endocarditis and vasculitis, and the toxic effects of alcohol. Additionally, drugs that depress myocardial contractility such as beta-blockers and nondihydropyridine CCBs may lead to heart failure.

(continues)

BACK TO THE BASICS (continued)

Restriction of ventricular filling may be caused by pericardial constriction or effusion, an atrial myxoma, mitral or tricuspid valvular stenosis, or increased ventricular stiffness as in ventricular hypertrophy, which is often a result of hypertension.

Although there are many causes of heart failure, hypertension is present in 75% of heart failure patients and 70% of cases are attributed to coronary heart disease. CHD now exceeds hypertension as the most common cause of heart failure. Heart failure can often be prevented by controlling other cardiovascular risk factors.

Pathophysiology of Heart Failure

Regardless of the cause of heart failure, several processes will occur in an effort to restore cardiac output. These compensatory responses include the following:

- Activation of the sympathetic nervous system in an effort to increase heart rate and contractility. Cardiac output is the product of heart rate and stroke volume, so it makes sense that increasing the heart rate or any of the factors that influence stroke volume—in this case contractility—will increase the cardiac output. Remember, stroke volume is influenced by preload, afterload, and contractility.

- Increasing preload is another means of increasing the stroke volume. When cardiac output declines, blood is redistributed to the most vital organs, the brain and heart, resulting in decreased renal perfusion. The kidney was designed to perceive a reduction in blood flow as a sign of reduced blood volume and will respond by activating the renin-angiotensin-aldosterone system. This results in sodium and water retention at the kidney in an effort to increase blood volume and, therefore, preload. When preload is increased, the increased blood volume stretches the ventricle muscle fibers. This stretch results in a more efficient muscle contraction, thereby increased cardiac output.

- Angiotensin II, which is activated by the kidney as just described, causes more vasoconstriction and further shunting of blood to vital organs.

These compensatory processes were designed to ensure blood flow to vital organs during acute drops in blood pressure or renal perfusion and are not ideal when activated for lengthy periods of time as in chronic heart failure. The negative effects of these processes when activated chronically include:

- Insufficient time for diastolic filling, which may actually worsen the cardiac output by decreasing preload. This is due to increased heart rate from sympathetic stimulation.

- Increased myocardial oxygen demand, which may precipitate or aggravate ischemia. This is due to increased sympathetic stimulation.

- Pulmonary congestion from fluid leaking out of the bloodstream into the alveoli. This occurs when the additional blood volume, which initially results in increased contractility, exceeds the oncotic pressure that holds the fluid in the vasculature.

- Increased afterload makes it harder for the heart to pump the blood into the arterial circulation and may worsen cardiac output. Afterload is increased because the vasoconstriction that shunts the blood to vital organs also constricts the arterial system.

- Remodeling is a detrimental process characterized by hypertrophy, fibrosis, and loss of myocytes, which alters the size, shape, and function of the ventricle. Many factors may lead to remodeling including an insult to the myocardium as in an infarction or mechanical changes such as the altered pressures and volumes encountered in cardiomyopathy. Remodeling affects the conduction system and valve function. Atrial stretch may provoke supraventricular arrhythmias. Remodeling of the ventricle may alter the conduction through the ventricle resulting in the development of left BBB or ventricular arrhythmias. This is why heart failure is associated with a rate of sudden death that is six to nine times that of the general public. Remodeling may also cause asynchronous ventricular contraction, which diminishes contractility. Also, valve dysfunction may occur because the altered shape of the heart alters the position and functionality of the valves.

Clinical Manifestations of Heart Failure

Left-sided heart failure, failure of the left ventricle, causes fluid to back up into the left atrium and into the pulmonary circulation. This typically manifests as dyspnea, fatigue, paroxysmal nocturnal dyspnea, orthopnea, and pulmonary edema. Pulmonary edema is characterized by a cough with wheezing and blood-tinged secretions, which look like pink, frothy sputa.

Patients with left ventricular failure may also complain of sudden weight gain; a frequent dry, hacking cough; loss of appetite; or fatigue. Physical exam may reveal basilar rales, pulmonary edema, an S3 gallop, or a pleural effusion.

Right-sided heart failure, failure of the right ventricle, causes the blood to back up into the right atrium, the vena cava, and to the periphery. Patients with right ventricular failure may complain of peripheral edema or GI problems such as abdominal pain, anorexia, nausea, and bloating. Physical exam findings include jugular venous distention, hepatojugular reflux, hepatomegaly, or edema.

Diagnosis

Although heart failure is often suspected by clinical presentation, a firm diagnosis of heart failure is difficult because there is no single test that will confirm the diagnosis. Labs can be useful in identifying cardiac risk factors and underlying causes that may cause or worsen heart failure. Useful labs include a complete blood count, serum electrolytes, liver function tests, creatinine, urinalysis, and a lipid profile. An EKG is ordered to assess for underlying cardiac conditions, but there are no specific EKG abnormalities associated with heart failure. A chest X-ray is useful in identifying an enlarged cardiac silhouette, pleural effusions, and pulmonary edema.

An echocardiogram is essential to identify any structural or valvular abnormalities, wall motion abnormalities, systolic or diastolic failure, and to determine the ejection fraction. Biochemical markers such as B-type natriuretic peptide (BNP) are increasingly being used in the management of heart failure. BNP is secreted in response to ventricular stretch and pressure overload, as part of the body's compensatory response in heart failure. Its function is to counteract the vasoconstriction that occurs as a compensatory mechanism in heart failure.

Serum BNP levels are reserved for differentiating the cause of dyspnea when it is unclear if a pulmonary or cardiac etiology exists. BNP levels are not useful in patients with end-stage renal disease or in patients who are taking Natrecor (nesiritide). False-negative results may occur in patients with acute pulmonary edema and heart failure due to mitral regurgitation.

Pearl

Patients with significant congestive heart failure have BNP levels greater than 400 pg/mL; cardiac dysfunction is highly unlikely to be the cause of dyspnea if the BNP level is less than 100 pg/mL. If the level is between 100 and 400 pg/mL, compensated left ventricular dysfunction, pulmonary embolism, or cor pulmonale may be the cause of dyspnea.

Pearl

If the BNP is less than 430 at time of discharge, the patient is less likely to be readmitted for another heart failure exacerbation.

Bottom Line	
BNP level	**Clinical scenario**
<100	Unlikely to have heart failure
0–200	May have pulmonary disease
>400	Significant heart failure likely

An ischemic evaluation with coronary arteriography or noninvasive imaging may be necessary if the patient has a history of CHD, angina, or ischemia unless the patient is not eligible for revascularization procedures. Some patients may require screening for sleep-disordered breathing, HIV, hemochromatosis, rheumatological diseases, amyloidosis, or pheochromocytoma if there is clinical suspicion of these illnesses or if the etiology of heart failure is unidentified.

Management

Early identification and management of risk factors is crucial to limiting the devastating and progressive nature of heart failure, both prior to and subsequent to establishing a diagnosis of heart failure.

Prevention of Heart Failure

Effective treatment of hypertension, diabetes, hyperlipidemia, obesity, and prevention of MI will reduce the risk of developing heart failure. Avoidance of excessive alcohol, tobacco use, certain illicit drugs, and cardiotoxic medications is also advisable. Valvular abnormalities also increase the risk of heart failure and should be appropriately managed.

Patients at risk for developing heart failure should be assessed for heart failure symptoms and undergo a screening EKG and CXR. If cardiomegaly, an S3 gallop, a potentially significant heart murmur, LVH, left BBB, or pathologic Q waves are identified, an echocardiogram is indicated. An echocardiogram should also be obtained in patients with underlying CHD, valvular disease, atrial fibrillation or flutter, or in those with a first-degree relative with cardiomyopathy.

ACE inhibitors are recommended for patients who are at a high risk of developing heart failure. This includes patients with a history of CHD, peripheral vascular disease, or stroke. Beta-blockers should be instituted in patients with a prior MI to reduce the risk of developing heart failure.

Lifestyle Modifications

Encourage the following lifestyle modifications among heart failure patients: weight reduction, smoking cessation, avoidance of alcohol and other cardiotoxic substances, exercise, sodium (and possibly fluid) restriction, and monitoring of daily weights. Individuals with heart failure should limit sodium intake to 2–3 g daily. More severe heart failure may require further reduction to less than 2 g daily.

If fluid restriction is necessary to limit episodic decompensation, limit water to 2 liters or 8 cups per day (64 ounces total). This includes all beverages and any water taken with medications.

Exercising by cycling or walking 3–5 days per week has been shown to reduce mortality and hospitalization in patients with heart failure and should be encouraged. Frequent outpatient monitoring is essential to reduce hospitalizations by timely identification of decompensation and early recognition of straying from the heart failure regimen.

> **Pearl**
>
> To keep track of how much fluid they are consuming each day, suggest that patients fill a 2-liter bottle with water each day. Patients should drink only from this container unless they dump out the amount of fluid they consumed from other sources.

Medications

ACE inhibitors and beta-blockers have been proven to improve mortality and interfere with the progression of heart failure. The combination of an ACE inhibitor and a beta-blocker is the cornerstone of medical therapy in heart failure.

ACE Inhibitors

ACE inhibitors have been shown to decrease mortality, reduce hospitalizations, improve symptoms, and improve exercise tolerance. They are first-line therapy for all patients with an EF less than or equal to 40%, regardless of whether symptoms are present.

ARBs

Studies have shown that ARBs have similar beneficial effects as ACE inhibitors and should be used if an ACE inhibitor is not tolerated.

> **Pearl**
>
> Patients with heart failure often require many medications, and it may take a few months to see results. Explain the benefits of each medication to patients so that they understand the need to remain on their regimen.

> **Pearl**
>
> Here's how I explain the merits of ACE inhibitors to patients:
>
> Fill a balloon with water and hold the opening closed with one hand. You can then use your free hand to squeeze the balloon and force water out of the opening. If you have weak hands and can't squeeze very much, lightening your grip on the opening of the balloon will allow the water to flow out of the balloon anyway.
>
> The same is true of the heart. If it is too weak to squeeze (or pump) very much, you can simply reduce the grip on the aorta so that blood can easily exit the heart. This is what ACE inhibitors do by relaxing the arterial circulation so that the heart doesn't have to overcome as much pressure in order to pump the blood forward.

Hydralazine and Oral Nitrates

If patients are unable to take an ACE inhibitor or ARB because of renal insufficiency or hyperkalemia, the combination of hydralazine and oral nitrates should be considered.

Also, all African Americans with NYHA class II through IV heart failure due to left ventricular systolic dysfunction should be placed on a combination of hydralazine and oral nitrates in addition to standard ACE inhibitor and beta-blocker therapy. This combination may also be considered in non-African Americans with left ventricular systolic dysfunction that remains symptomatic despite the use of ACE inhibitors and other appropriate therapy.

Beta-Blockers

All patients with an EF less than or equal to 40% should be placed on a beta-blocker along with an ACE inhibitor unless contraindicated. The beta-blockers bisoprolol (Zebeta), carvedilol (Coreg), and long-acting metoprolol (Toprol XL) have been shown to decrease heart failure symptoms and to decrease hospitalizations and mortality rates. Patients admitted with decompensated heart failure should begin beta-blocker therapy once their volume status is optimized and they no longer require IV diuretics or inotropic support. Beta-blockers should be continued during exacerbations of heart failure, but a temporary reduction of dose may be considered. Avoid abrupt discontinuation of beta-blockers.

Beta-blockers are often well tolerated and, therefore, recommended in heart failure patients with concomitant diabetes, COPD, and peripheral vascular disease. Caution is required if patients have had recurrent hypoglycemia, asthma, or resting limb ischemia. Avoid beta-blockers in profound bradycardia, profound hypotension, and asthmatics with active bronchospasm.

Aldosterone Antagonists

Aldosterone blockers are recommended in addition to standard therapy in all patients with an EF of less than or equal to 35% and NYHA class III or IV heart failure. They are also recommended in post-MI patients with an EF less than or equal to 40% and heart failure symptoms despite appropriate therapy.

Aldosterone antagonists should be avoided in significant renal dysfunction (creatinine should be less than or equal to 2.5 mg/dL in men and less than or equal to 2.0 mg/dL in women) or hyperkalemia (potassium should be less than or equal to 5.0 mEq/L). Monitoring of serum potassium levels should be performed frequently after initiation or change in dosage.

Bottom Line

When prescribing beta-blockers in heart failure, "start low and go slow." Titrate to the highest dose tolerated. Bisoprolol (Zebeta): starting dose 2.5–5 mg once daily orally; target dose 10 mg once daily. Carvedilol (Coreg): starting dose 3.125 mg twice daily orally; target dose 25 mg twice daily. Metoprolol succinate (Toprol XL): starting dose 12.5–25 mg once daily orally; target dose 200 mg once daily.

Digoxin

Long-term digoxin therapy has been shown to reduce symptoms, increase exercise tolerance, decrease the risk of heart failure progression, reduce hospitalization for decompensated heart failure, and control ventricular rate in atrial fibrillation.

Digoxin does not improve survival and is therefore used only as an adjunct to ACE inhibitors, diuretics, and beta-blockers in class II–IV heart failure.

A digoxin level less than 1.0 ng/ mL is effective and a dose of 0.125 is usually sufficient.

Diuretics

Diuretics are used to relieve the fluid overload and congestive symptoms that often accompany heart failure. If patients are not fluid overloaded, you can omit this class of medications. Loop diuretics are the most effective in the treatment of heart failure and should be titrated to achieve euvolemia. Increasing the frequency of dosing to two or three times daily provides more effective diuresis than larger single doses.

IV diuretics or the addition of metolazone (Zaroxolyn) may be required periodically. Monitor volume status and electrolytes closely when these are required.

Anticoagulants and Antiplatelets

Chronic anticoagulation with warfarin (Coumadin) is indicated in chronic atrial fibrillation, a known thrombus, or for 3 months following a large MI that has caused ischemic cardiomyopathy. It is controversial in heart failure unless one of these comorbidities is present, but may be considered in patients with a dilated cardiomyopathy with an EF less than 35%.

Aspirin is recommended in patients with heart failure only when due to ischemic cardiomyopathy. Higher doses may worsen heart failure, so 75 or 81 mg doses are recommended.

Vasodilators

Vasodilators provide symptomatic improvement by decreasing preload and reducing cardiac-filling pressures. Nitrates and nesiritide (Natrecor) are examples.

Inotropes

Positive inotropic agents are often used in the treatment of patients with acute decompensated heart failure. Several studies have shown that dobutamine and milrinone are associated with an increased risk of arrhythmias and that they may increase mortality, particularly in patients with ischemic heart failure. These medications should not be routinely used in patients with acute heart failure, but reserved for patients with low cardiac output.

Levosimendan is an inotropic agent, which has been shown to provide hemodynamic improvement in patients with acute decompensated heart failure. It is not associated with arrhythmias and may be associated with improved mortality compared with dobutamine.

Device Therapy

Implantable Cardioverter-Defibrillator

Patients with NYHA class II to III symptoms and an EF of 30–35% or less should be considered for an implantable cardioverter-defibrillator (ICD) regardless of whether they have CHD. If patients have chronic, severe refractory heart failure with no reasonable expectation for improvement, then ICD implantation is not recommended.

Cardiac Resynchronization Therapy

A prolonged QRS duration indicates inefficient contraction of the ventricles. In patients with severe heart failure, every bit of blood ejected is crucial to maintaining cardiac output. Therefore, cohesive conduction is often essential in such patients. In patients with advanced heart failure and a prolonged QRS interval, cardiac-resynchronization therapy (CRT) decreases the combined risk of death from any cause.

CRT involves insertion of a biventricular pacemaker. A typical pacemaker has a ventricular lead only in the left ventricle. A biventricular pacemaker places leads in both ventricles, allowing stimulation of both the right and left ventricles simultaneously. This results in a cohesive contraction of both chambers, thereby increasing the cardiac output.

CRT should be considered in individuals with moderate to severe heart failure (NYHA class III/IV) with an EF less than or equal to 35% who are symptomatic despite optimal medical therapy and have a QRS duration of 120 ms or longer. If the patient also meets criteria for an ICD, a biventricular ICD can be placed instead of a biventricular pacemaker.

Surgical Therapy

In patients with severe, end-stage heart failure, surgical procedures may need to be considered. Oftentimes, this means simply referring the patient to a major center where more advanced procedures are performed. Surgical options include a cardiomyoplasty, ventriculectomy, heart transplantation, or placement of a ventricular-assist device.

Vaccinations

Influenza and pneumococcal vaccinations are recommended in all heart failure patients.

Medications to Avoid in Heart Failure

Some medications may worsen heart failure or induce an exacerbation. Take the time to ensure patients are only on the following medications if the benefits outweigh the risks.

- Most antiarrhythmics: Only amiodarone and dofetilide should be used in heart failure because they have been shown not to worsen survival. If amiodarone is added, reduce the dose of other agents such as warfarin, digoxin, and statins and monitor for possible drug interactions.
- Nondihydropyridine CCBs
- NSAIDS and COX-2 inhibitors
- Thiazolidinediones should not be used in patients recovering from STEMI who have New York Heart Association class III or IV heart failure
- Certain chemotherapeutic agents

Patient Visits

Heart failure management is complex and differs based on whether patients are presenting for the first time and whether they are symptomatic, asymptomatic, acutely decompensated, or end stage. Each of these scenarios and the recommended approach to the patient are covered here.

The Initial Assessment of Heart Failure

History and Physical

When seeing a heart failure patient for the first time, it is important to perform a thorough history and physical. Ensure the patient is on all beneficial medications. Note whether the patient is on any medications, OTC, or alternative products that may be contributing to their heart failure. Inquire about use of tobacco, alcohol, and illicit drugs, which all may cause cardiotoxicity.

Obtain orthostatic BP measurements, weight, and BMI or waist-to-hip ratio. Assess the patient's volume status by noting the presence of jugular venous distension, ascites, hepatomegaly, hepatojugular reflux, pulmonary rales, and/or dependent edema. Seek out underlying causes and screen for cardiac risk factors.

Diagnostic Studies

The following studies may be considered on an individual basis:

- Complete blood count
- Urinalysis
- Electrolytes including magnesium and calcium
- BUN/Cr
- TSH level
- Fasting glucose level
- Glycosylated hemoglobin (HG A1C)
- Fasting lipid panel
- Liver function tests
- Albumen level
- BNP level (if the diagnosis of CHF is uncertain)
- EKG
- Chest radiograph
- Echocardiogram
- Ischemic evaluation with cardiac catheterization or noninvasive imaging
- Screening for sleep-disordered breathing, HIV, hemochromatosis, rheumatological diseases, amyloidosis, or pheochromocytoma

Management

Provide patient education regarding heart failure and how patients can self-manage this chronic disease by checking and recording daily weights, restricting sodium intake, and observing their own fluid status. There are some wonderful programs to help you cover this information with your patients efficiently such as HeartSteps offered by Lincare. Many hospitals have a heart failure nurse hotline that is available for free when patients are discharged from the hospital with a diagnosis of heart failure.

Heart Failure Follow-up Visits

History and Physical

When performing a follow-up visit on a patient with heart failure, identify any current symptoms indicative of a heart failure exacerbation. Specifically, ask about sudden weight gain, dyspnea, orthopnea, PND, increased dependent edema, abdominal bloating, dry hacking cough, or increased fatigue. Ask the patient if he or she is checking weight daily and review the weight record with them. If necessary, reinforce the benefits of this simple means of preventing morbidity. Identify any signs of volume overload on physical examination as discussed previously.

If the patient exhibits any signs or symptoms of fluid overload, inquire about any dietary indiscretions (sodium or fluid intake), medications, tobacco, alcohol, illicit drugs, chemotherapeutic agents, or alternative therapies that may have contributed to the exacerbation.

If patients are experiencing exertional dyspnea, ask them how much activity results in symptoms; for instance, do they become short of breath walking from room to room, from the parking lot to your office, or walking up stairs. Use this information to determine their NYHA functional class.

If patients are short of breath at rest or with minimal activity, assess their ability to perform activities of daily living (ADLs) and desired activities.

Diagnostic Studies

- Electrolytes (particularly potassium levels) and renal function should be monitored routinely in patients with chronic heart failure.
- Routine evaluation of the ejection fraction in clinically stable patients is not necessary.

Management

Make sure the patient is taking all recommended medications unless contraindicated or not tolerated. Make sure no cardiotoxic medications are given unless the benefits outweigh the detriments.

Pearl

Eating out is another way that patients become decompensated. Restaurants often prepare meals with more salt than a home-cooked meal. Sometimes you may even need to be wary of home cooking. A young woman with severe cardiomyopathy learned, after several admissions for decompensated heart failure, that she cannot eat meals prepared by well-meaning friends.

All patients with a reduced ejection fraction should be on an ACE inhibitor and beta-blocker regardless of whether they have had an MI or are symptomatic. Titrate both to the highest tolerable doses during each follow-up visit. If the patient is intolerant of the ACE inhibitor, an ARB may be substituted.

If the patient is symptomatic, reinforce dietary restrictions and add or increase a diuretic. Loop diuretics such as furosemide (Lasix) are preferred and typically require potassium supplementation. Note that patients with renal failure or those taking ACE inhibitors, ARBs, or aldosterone antagonists may not require potassium supplementation. Patients with excessive weight gain or marked symptoms may require hospitalization and more aggressive management as discussed later.

An aldosterone antagonist should be added to the regimen if the patient has moderately severe or severe symptoms. Digoxin and/or the combination of hydralazine with an oral nitrate may be beneficial additions if the patient is still symptomatic despite appropriate use of the above medications.

Pearl

Of the beta-blockers, only bisoprolol (Zebeta), carvedilol (Coreg), and sustained release metoprolol (Toprol XL) have proven mortality reduction in heart failure.

Stage 1	No limitation
Stage 2	Slight limitation; symptoms occur with ordinary activity such as walking up a flight of stairs
Stage 3	Marked limitation; symptoms occur with less-than-ordinary activity such as walking from room to room
Stage 4	Severe limitation; symptoms occur with minimal activity, such as getting dressed, or at rest

FIGURE 20.1 NYHA Functional Classification of Heart Disease

Review the criteria for cardiac-resynchronization therapy and/or ICD implantation to determine if the patient should be considered for such devices.

Schedule close follow-up visits in an effort to avoid clinical deterioration by timely identification of communication errors or nonadherence to the medical regimen. Patients with heart failure have shown reduced hospital admissions if they are enrolled in a heart failure clinic.

Acute Decompensation of Heart Failure

History and Physical

Patients with acute decompensation of heart failure typically present with signs and symptoms of congestion and volume overload. Far less commonly, patients may present with hypotension and poor renal or other end-organ perfusion due to severe left ventricular systolic dysfunction.

Diagnostic Studies

Acute decompensation of heart failure is diagnosed by clinical findings. If the diagnosis is uncertain, a chest radiograph or BNP level may be helpful. Weight should be monitored daily and electrolytes, including magnesium, and renal function should be followed closely. If the patient requires admission, strict measurement of fluid intake and output should be ordered.

Management

The first priority in managing acute decompensation of heart failure is determining whether to admit the patient. Hospital admission is recommended if patients present with hypotension, declining renal function, altered mental status, resting tachypnea, or hypoxia. Admission is also essential in patients with acute coronary syndrome and a hemodynamically significant arrhythmia including new onset rapid atrial fibrillation. Patients may be considered for admission if they have a weight gain of 5 or more kilograms or congestive signs or symptoms, particularly if there is no prior history of heart failure. Patients with repeated ICD discharges, a major electrolyte disturbance, or concomitant stroke, transient ischemic attack, diabetic ketoacidosis, pneumonia, or pulmonary embolus should all be considered for admission.

Precipitating factors should be identified and discussed with all patients who have had a heart failure exacerbation regardless of whether admission is required. Common precipitators include dietary indiscretions, medication nonadherence, arrhythmias, hypertensive exacerbation, myocardial ischemia/infarct, anemia, or a thyroid abnormality.

Management should include sodium and fluid restriction. Loop diuretics are typically given intravenously. If congestion fails to improve, consider increasing the dose, adding metolazone (Zaroxolyn) or spironolactone or renal dialysis. IV vasodilators such as nesiritide (Natrecor), nitroglycerine, or sodium nitroprusside may be added to diuretics for rapid relief of congestive symptoms and are recommended when severe hypertension or pulmonary edema is present. Vasodilators should not be used if patients are hypotensive. Positive inotropes should be used scarcely.

End-Stage, Refractory Heart Failure

Each year, more than 40,000 patients with heart failure progress to the end stage of disease. When patients become refractory to all appropriate treatment and have persistent symptoms at rest, patients are considered end stage.

These patients require careful management of volume status with strict dietary restriction of salt and fluids. Patients should be enrolled in a heart failure program and be advised of the importance of daily weight measurements.

If the patient may be eligible for cardiac transplantation, refer the patient to an appropriate center for evaluation. A left ventricular assist device may be considered for therapeutic purposes or as a bridge to transplantation.

End-of-life care should be discussed with the patient and family. They should be made aware of the patient's prognosis and discussion about resuscitation, advanced directives, and the option of inactivating an ICD should be facilitated. The patient's wishes should be reassessed frequently to ensure they have not changed. Information regarding available hospice services should be provided as well.

In addition to standard heart failure therapy, end-stage patients may require vasodilator (nesiritide [Natrecor]) or positive inotrope (dobutamine or milrinone) infusion for palliation of symptoms. Inotropic medications may be useful in allowing patients to be discharged to die in the comfort of their home, but they should only be used as a last resort as they increase mortality.

Opiates should be provided for relief of pain and dyspnea and patients should be screened, and managed, for depression.

Diastolic Heart Failure

Discussions of heart failure usually refer to systolic dysfunction; however, up to 40% of patients with heart failure have diastolic dysfunction rather than systolic dysfunction. Causes of diastolic dysfunction include coronary heart disease, hypertension, aging, diabetes mellitus, obesity, and aortic stenosis.

Distinguishing diastolic from systolic dysfunction is essential because they are managed differently. Because the presentation is similar to that of systolic failure, echocardiography is the best noninvasive means of diagnosis.

Treatment of diastolic dysfunction includes addressing any underlying causes and decreasing left ventricular–filling pressure without decreasing cardiac output. Maintaining atrial-ventricular synchrony and sinus rhythm often improves clinical function. Treatment of diastolic dysfunction includes the use of CCBs, beta-blockers, and ACE inhibitors. Because diastolic dysfunction is caused by the inability of the ventricle to fill adequately, exercise caution when using diuretics and nitrates because these medications also reduce preload and may worsen the dysfunction. Diuretics may be used cautiously for pulmonary congestion and nitrates may be used cautiously in the presence of concomitant myocardial ischemia. Positive inotropic or chronotropic agents, potent vasodilators, and alpha-blockers should be avoided because they can worsen diastolic function when systolic function is normal.

Chapter 21

Atrial Fibrillation

Introduction

Atrial fibrillation (AF) is the most common sustained rhythm disturbance encountered in clinical practice. AF is commonly associated with other cardiovascular conditions and advancing age, so naturally, the prevalence of AF has increased as survival rates from other cardiovascular conditions have improved and the population has begun to age.

Pearl

Blood clots are most often located in the left atrial appendage (LAA), an area that is not adequately visualized by a standard transthoracic echocardiogram (TTE). For this reason, a transesophageal echocardiogram (TEE) is used to look for the presence of clots in the LAA.

Hemodynamic impairment and thromboembolism are responsible for most morbidity and mortality attributed to AF. Hemodynamic changes that result from AF include the loss of a synchronized atrial contraction, also known as the *atrial kick*. The additional blood that would have been squeezed into the ventricle if a normal atrial contraction had been present is small, but often essential in patients with reduced cardiac output. Heart failure patients may require synchronized atrial contraction for improved functional ability. Hemodynamic compromise may also result from a rapid ventricular rate. Rapid ventricular rates in AF may also cause cardiomyopathy, which is reversible once adequate rate control is achieved.

Ineffective contraction of the atrium may cause blood to remain stagnant in the atrium, leading to clot formation and the possibility of thromboembolism. Ischemic stroke occurs in 5% of patients with nonvalvular AF per year. The annual risk of stroke increases dramatically with advancing age. While patients in their 50s have about a 1.5% chance of stroke, 23.5% of patients in their 80s are at risk of stroke.

Etiology

Advanced age, concomitant cardiovascular conditions, and the presence of cardiovascular risk factors increase the chance of developing AF. Hypertension, valvular heart disease, and heart failure are the greatest risk factors for the development of AF. Patients with a history of MI, diabetes, cigarette smoking, or EKG evidence of LVH also have an increased risk of AF.

AF is associated with underlying heart disease because such conditions often cause structural changes that distort the atrium (i.e., dilatation, hypertrophy, fibrosis, inflammation), which may alter its electrical properties.

AF may be precipitated by anything that increases sympathetic stimulation such as hyperthyroidism, anxiety, electrocution, or a pheochromocytoma. Caffeine, alcohol, or sympathomimetic drugs may also increase sympathetic stimulation resulting in AF. Increased vagal tone, such as during sleep, after a large meal, or with the use of digoxin or beta-blockers, has also been shown to precipitate AF.

Pulmonary disorders such as pulmonary embolus, bronchopneumonia, or bronchial carcinoma may predispose patients to AF.

Inflammatory disorders that affect the heart may lead to AF. These include pericarditis, amyloidosis, myocarditis, and lupus. If a primary or secondary cancer occurs in the atrium, AF may ensue.

Patients who are young (under 60 years of age) and develop AF in the absence of clinical or echocardiographic evidence of underlying heart disease or other identifiable causes are said to have lone AF. They have a good prognosis.

Classification

If the patient is diagnosed with AF for the first time, it is simply called first-detected AF. Subsequent episodes of AF that last longer than 30 seconds and have no reversible cause are classified based on how long they last and whether they terminate spontaneously. Episodes that have reversible causes are not classified, because it is unlikely that they will recur once the precipitating cause is removed.

Paroxysmal AF refers to episodic AF that spontaneously resolves. Persistent AF refers to sustained AF that requires treatment to resolve. These patients may be successfully converted to sinus rhythm with antiarrhythmic medications or electrical cardioversion. Permanent AF refers to long-standing AF (greater than 1 year).

Clinical Presentation

Some patients may remain asymptomatic. Others may describe palpitations, irregular heartbeats, tachycardia, chest discomfort, dyspnea, weakness, lightheadedness, or syncope.

If patients have vagally mediated AF, they may perceive an irregular heart beat, but rarely complain of dyspnea, dizziness, or syncope.

Diagnosis

AF is diagnosed by capturing the irregular rhythm on EKG. If the patient presents with symptoms consistent with AF but are in sinus rhythm during the evaluation, a Holter monitor, event monitor, or continuous telemetry monitoring may identify the rhythm disturbance later.

A rhythm strip that includes both the onset and termination of the arrhythmia is helpful in differentiating AF from other rhythm disturbances. If the onset and termination are abrupt, the rhythm is most likely AF or some other form of SVT. If the onset and termination are gradual, it may actually be sinus tachycardia.

If the patient has a pacemaker, you may need to disable the device in order to view the patient's underlying rhythm. The atria may still be fibrillating in these patients, even if they have a regularly paced ventricular rhythm. Therefore, they are still at risk of stroke and, depending on the functionality of their AV node, rapid ventricular rate.

> **Pearl**
> When presenting a patient to your supervising physician in order to diagnose an arrhythmia, have a rhythm strip or EKG that captures the onset and termination of the arrhythmia whenever possible.

Management

Management of AF may seem complex, but can be simplified by breaking it down into the following four objectives:

1. Identify underlying conditions or precipitators.
2. Ensure adequate control of the ventricular rate.
3. Minimize the risk of stroke.
4. Determine whether restoration of sinus rhythm is warranted and how to accomplish this.

Underlying Conditions and Precipitators

Correctly managing reversible causes of AF often will resolve the dysrhythmia and with avoidance of such triggers, the patient is unlikely to have recurrences of AF. Advise the patient to avoid caffeine, OTC products containing pseudoephedrine or other sympathomimetics, alcohol, and tobacco.

Because HTN is the most important risk factor for ischemic stroke, it is vital that HTN is adequately controlled in patients with AF and concomitant HTN.

Thyroid, liver, and kidney function should be evaluated along with hemoglobin and electrolytes to rule out any precipitating factors.

A chest X-ray is indicated to evaluate for possible pulmonary pathology.

An echocardiogram will identify any structural abnormalities, valvular abnormalities, infiltrative diseases, or malignancies.

An ischemic evaluation (i.e., a stress test or cardiac catheterization) may be warranted if the clinical presentation and risk-factor profile suggest the possibility of underlying ischemia. A cardiac catheterization would be reserved for very high-risk patients, of course.

> **Bottom Line**
>
> Order a CBC, BMP, LFTs, TSH level, chest radiograph, echocardiogram, and consider an ischemic evaluation.

> **Pearl**
>
> Some patients have tachy-brady syndrome, which means that the rate is sometimes fast and sometimes slow. Management of tachy-brady syndrome often requires a pacemaker to prevent bradycardia and then AV nodal blockers can be added to prevent tachycardia.

Rate Control

Patients with AF may have fast, slow, or normal ventricular rates. The ventricular response depends on the ability of the AV node to conduct as well as the patient's vagal and sympathetic tone.

Beta-blockers, nondihydropyridine CCBs, and digoxin are the most commonly employed agents for rate control in AF. Diltiazem (Cardizem, Dilacor, Tiazac) and verapamil (Calan, Isoptin) are nondihydropyridine CCBs that are effective at lowering heart rate. They are often given via IV for rapid reduction in heart rate as they act within minutes.

Beta-blockers are also useful in IV form and are the agents of choice for rate control in patients with catecholamine-driven AF as in thyrotoxicosis.

In patients with heart failure, IV digoxin may also be considered for rate control. Digoxin is effective at controlling ventricular rate at rest, but with sympathetic stimulation, as in exertion, this medication is overridden and tachycardia may result. For this reason, digoxin is usually reserved for sedentary patients.

> **For Example**
> Give a bolus of diltiazem 0.25 mg/kg IV over 2 minutes followed by an infusion of 5 to 15 mg/hr to keep the heart rate below 120, keeping systolic BP greater than 100.

In addition to acute management of rapid ventricular rate, beta-blockers, CCBs, and digoxin can also be administered orally for chronic ventricular rate control. Amiodarone can be used as a last resort for rate control when other measures are ineffective.

Ablation of the AV node is an acceptable alternative to pharmacological therapy if medications are not tolerated or are ineffective at controlling the heart rate. If cardiomyopathy has resulted from tachycardia, ablation may be necessary. Ablation should only be performed for rate control once pharmacological control has been attempted.

> **Caution**
> In patients with an accessory pathway such as Wolff-Parkinson-White, avoid giving medications that slow conduction through the AV node (digoxin, beta-blockers, CCBs) while patients are tachycardic. These medications will block conduction through the AV node, which may result in increased conduction down the accessory pathway. This can cause a rapid ventricular response that may degenerate into ventricular fibrillation and sudden cardiac death. Suspect an accessory pathway if the ventricular rate is greater than 200 bpm.
>
> Treatment in these cases is accomplished by cardioversion either electrically or with amiodarone or type I antiarrhythmic agents, such as IV ibutilide or procainamide. Oral beta-blockers or CCBs can then be used for maintenance therapy.

CVA Prophylaxis

The following recommendations for stroke prophylaxis apply to patients with paroxysmal, persistent, or permanent AF as well as for atrial flutter.

Unless contraindicated, antithrombotic therapy is recommended for all patients with AF other than those with lone AF. In lone AF (patients less than 60 years of age without heart disease or risk factors for thromboembolism) long-term anticoagulation is not recommended with warfarin (Coumadin). Because the risk of thromboembolism is low, aspirin has not yet been shown to outweigh the risks of bleeding in these patients either.

Aspirin is a reasonable alternative to warfarin in low risk patients. Patients are considered to be low risk for embolic stroke if they have *only one* of the following:

- Age greater than or equal to 75 years
- Hypertension
- Heart failure or impaired left ventricular function
- Diabetes mellitus

In patients with *more than one* of these risk factors for stroke, warfarin use is recommended. Additionally, patients at the highest risk for stroke, those with a prior history of thromboembolism, rheumatic mitral stenosis, or a mechanical heart valve, should be placed on warfarin therapy.

When using warfarin, the target international normalized ratio (INR) is 2.0 to 3.0 except in those with mechanical heart valves where the target INR is 2.5–3.5. In patients 75 years of age or older or with tolerability issues, it is acceptable to treat to an INR of 1.6–2.5.

Pearl

Discuss treatment options with the patient and allow them to participate in the decision making regarding the use of warfarin. Weigh the individual patient's risk of stroke versus bleeding and consider the patient's preference and ability to comply with warfarin monitoring.

Pearl

It is reasonable to hold warfarin for surgical or diagnostic procedures for up to 1 week without administering heparin as long as the patient does not have a mechanical heart valve. If the procedure requires holding warfarin for longer than 1 week, heparin or low-molecular weight heparin (Lovenox) should be considered in high-risk patients.

Pearl

Patients with AF who have undergone percutaneous coronary intervention or revascularization surgery should receive low-dose aspirin (less than 100 mg) and/or clopidogrel (Plavix) in addition to warfarin. Following stent implantation, patients should remain on low-dose aspirin and clopidogrel in addition to warfarin therapy. Monitor therapy very closely while the patient remains on other antithrombotic medications.

BACK TO THE BASICS

There are four classes of antiarrhythmic drugs based on the primary effect the agent has on the action potential (Vaughan Williams Classification). The action potential is the electrical activity that occurs in the cells of muscles or nerves in response to mechanical, chemical, or electrical stimulation. Channels in the cardiac cell membrane open and close at different times during the action potential allowing ions (Na^+, K^+, Ca^{++}) to pass through the cell membrane and create a current.

Class 1 agents block sodium channels. Class 2 agents, the beta-blockers, inhibit the sympathetic nervous system. Class 3 agents prolong the duration of the action potential. Class 4 agents are CCBs (remember that calcium is needed to stimulate the contractile elements in the heart). Some medications may exert more than one of these effects or have metabolites that exert a different class of action.

Quinidine, procainamide (Pronestyl), and disopyramide (Norpace) are examples of class Ia antiarrhythmics. These agents have fallen out of favor due to excess toxicity; they all may cause torsades de pointes due to QT prolongation. Procainamide causes a lupus-like syndrome in up to 30% of patients. Disopyramide causes significant anticholinergic side effects and may worsen heart failure. Lidocaine is an example of a class Ib agent. It is administered intravenously due to its short half-life.

Flecainide (Tambocor) and propafenone (Rythmol) are class 1c agents. They suppress ventricular arrhythmias and are effective in preventing episodes of PSVT or atrial fibrillation. Class 1c agents should be avoided in patients with underlying heart disease such as coronary heart disease or congestive heart

(continues)

BACK TO THE BASICS (continued)

Pearl

To ensure the selection of the safest and least toxic antiarrhythmic agent, an echocardiogram and an ischemic evaluation is performed to assess for underlying ischemia or structural heart disease.

failure because of an increased risk of proarrhythmia and increased mortality rates in this setting. These agents may also cause slow atrial flutter with the possibility of a rapid ventricular response. To prevent this possibility, an AV nodal blocker (beta blocker, nondihydropyridine CCB, or digoxin) must be administered concomitantly.

The beta-blockers propranolol (Inderal), acebutolol (Sectral), and esmolol (Brevibloc) are class 2 agents indicated for the treatment of arrhythmias. Esmolol is often used after surgery to control ventricular rate in AF and atrial flutter. It is administered intravenously.

Class 3 agents include sotalol (Betapace), dofetilide (Tikosyn), amiodarone (Cordarone, Pacerone), bretylium, and ibutilide. Sotalol (Betapace) and dofetilide (Tikosyn) both function by prolonging the QT interval. Sotalol is a nonselective beta-blocker categorized as a class 3 antiarrhythmic. It is used for AF as well as for ventricular arrhythmias. Dofetilide has many drug interactions and must be administered with caution. These agents should be avoided in patients with heart failure.

Amiodarone is indicated for the prevention and treatment of ventricular fibrillation and recurrent hemodynamically destabilizing ventricular tachycardia. It is also the drug of choice in cardiac arrest. Although not FDA approved for AF, amiodarone is the most effective antiarrhythmic for preventing recurrences of AF and can convert AF to sinus rhythm.

Patients on amiodarone must be closely monitored for adverse reactions such as pulmonary fibrosis, thyroid dysfunction, hepatic necrosis, and optic neuritis. Baseline thyroid function tests, liver function tests, and a chest X-ray should be obtained and repeated every 3 to 6 months. Patients should also be reminded to have an annual eye exam. Although these adverse effects may occur at the 200 mg daily dose commonly used for AF, they are more common with higher doses such as the 400 mg daily dose used for ventricular arrhythmias. Amiodarone may also cause GI upset, skin reactions such as a blue-gray discoloration, bradyarrhythmias, and peripheral neuropathy. Because of toxicity issues, other antiarrhythmics are commonly employed first line. Amiodarone is typically reserved for patients with underlying structural heart disease or congestive heart failure who are prone to higher mortality rates with the use of other antiarrhythmics.

When instituting amiodarone, it is important to reduce the dose of digoxin and check a digoxin level soon afterward. This is because amiodarone can increase serum concentrations of digoxin, leading to potential toxicity. Amiodarone also potentiates the effect of beta-blockers, some CCBs, warfarin, and other antiarrhythmics.

The nondihydropyridine CCBs (verapamil and diltiazem) are class 4 agents. They are discussed in detail in Chapter 5.

Adenosine is a metabolite of persantine, which is often used for cardiac stress testing because of its short half-life and vasodilatation properties. It is not classified according to the Vaughn Williams Classification scheme, but is preferred over the CCBs for conversion of SVT.

Restoring Sinus Rhythm

Sinus rhythm can be restored by medications, electrical cardioversion, or non-invasive or invasive procedures. Because of high rates of failed cardioversion and of relapse, medications are often used in conjunction with electrical cardioversion to improve the odds of the patient converting to, and remaining in, sinus rhythm.

Anticoagulation During Cardioversion

Whenever sinus rhythm is restored, there is a risk of thromboembolic events. Because it usually takes about 48 hours of AF for a blood clot to form in the atrium, anticoagulation is recommended in all patients who have been in AF for at least 48 hours or if the duration is unknown. The patient's individualized risk of thromboembolism should be considered to determine whether anticoagulation is beneficial in patients who have been in AF for less than 48 hours.

A therapeutic level of warfarin is recommended for a minimum of 3 weeks prior to, and 4 weeks subsequent to, electrical or pharmacological cardioversion. If cardioversion needs to be performed urgently due to hemodynamic instability, a bolus of IV heparin followed by heparin infusion can be administered. A transesophageal echocardiogram (TEE) is useful to ensure that no left atrial or left atrial appendage thrombus is visualized. In either case, warfarin should still be given for 4 weeks after cardioversion because atrial stunning, which is associated with cardioversion, is associated with a high rate of thromboembolic events and resolves within several weeks of the procedure.

Choosing a Means of Cardioversion

When choosing an agent to restore sinus rhythm, consider how the patient's comorbidities may affect the agent's safety profile as well as the agent's efficacy in both converting to and maintaining sinus rhythm.

Electrical Cardioversion

Direct-current (electrical) cardioversion is indicated if the patient has a rapid ventricular rate in the setting of ischemia, symptomatic hypotension, heart failure, hemodynamic instability, or preexcitation with a very rapid rate. Electrical cardioversion may also be considered if patients have bothersome symptoms or if the patient prefers this approach. It is not recommended that electrical cardioversion be repeated frequently and it is contraindicated in hypokalemia or digoxin toxicity.

Propafenone, flecainide, ibutilide, sotalol, and amiodarone are all acceptable for pretreatment to improve the chances for successful cardioversion as well as to reduce the likelihood of relapse, especially in patients who have previously relapsed to AF after undergoing successful electrical cardioversion.

Pearl

Antiarrhythmic medications may cause atrial flutter with a rapid ventricular rate. To prevent the possibility of tachyarrhythmia, all patients who are placed on antiarrhythmic medications should be placed on a beta-blocker or nondihydropyridine CCB prior to initiation of an antiarrhythmic.

Pharmacological Cardioversion

According to guidelines published by the American Heart Association, propafenone (Rythmol), flecainide (Tambocor), dofetilide, and ibutilide are first-line agents for pharmacological cardioversion of AF. Of these, inpatient initiation is only recommended for dofetilide. Amiodarone is an acceptable alternative and can also be initiated as an outpatient.

Digoxin and sotalol are considered harmful when used for cardioversion and should not be used for this purpose.

Catheter ablation may be considered in patients who fail to respond to antiarrhythmic therapy.

Rate Versus Rhythm

The debate regarding the superiority of rate control versus restoration of sinus rhythm is currently a hot topic. The debate was sparked by the results of the AFFIRM trial which enrolled only minimally symptomatic or asymptomatic patients who were of advanced age or had another risk factor for stroke. The outcome of the trial was that there was no difference in quality of life, risk of stroke, or mortality regardless of whether patients were restored to sinus rhythm or not.

This study demonstrated that in older patients who remain asymptomatic on rate control medications, restoration of sinus rhythm is often unwarranted. However, it failed to address patients who were symptomatic despite adequate rate control. These patients may have improved quality of life with restoration of sinus rhythm and, therefore, it is considered appropriate to attempt restoration of sinus rhythm in these patients.

Additionally, the adage "atrial fibrillation begets atrial fibrillation" should apply to your decision making. If someone has been in AF for a long time, it may be nearly impossible to restore sinus rhythm. Hence, if you are considering rate control versus restoration of sinus rhythm in younger patients, remember that you may never be able to restore sinus rhythm years later if you do not restore it now. Young patients with a properly functioning left ventricle may do just as well with rate control as with restoration of sinus rhythm in the near future. However, if these patients develop heart failure many years later, they may require the "atrial kick" to improve their functional class. At this later date, restoration of sinus rhythm may be impossible.

Many factors are involved in the decision making regarding AF, thus necessitating an individualized approach to management. Current guidelines recommend that patients who remain symptomatic despite adequate rate control may be considered for restoration of sinus rhythm. Additionally, they suggest that in younger patients, especially those with lone AF, rhythm control may be preferable to rate control. They also suggest that it is acceptable to manage older patients who are asymptomatic without restoration of sinus rhythm.

Regardless of whether the patient is managed with rate control or restoration of sinus rhythm, anticoagulation is recommended.

Maintaining Sinus Rhythm

Recurrence of AF is common and many patients require prophylactic antiarrhythmic therapy. Underlying heart disease and female gender increase the probability of frequent recurrence. Patients with postoperative AF or those with a reversible cause, however, are unlikely to have a recurrence and do not need to be considered for prophylactic therapy. When deciding on a pharmacological agent for the maintenance of sinus rhythm, you will need to consider the patient's comorbidities.

In lone AF, propafenone, flecainide, and sotalol are first-line agents. In patients with concomitant heart failure, amiodarone or dofetilide are safest. Sotalol is the preferred agent in patients with concomitant CHD with amiodarone as a second-line agent. Amiodarone is the recommended agent in patients with substantial LVH, but propafenone and flecainide are preferred if LVH is mild because of their lower toxicities.

Catheter ablation of the pulmonary vein or the AV node is an alternative means of maintaining sinus rhythm. If the AV node is ablated, a pacemaker is required because there will be no conduction of impulses from the atrium to the ventricle once the AV node is ablated.

The indications for surgical management of AF are still evolving. The maze procedure significantly improves quality of life in patients with drug-refractory AF and has impressive results in maintaining sinus rhythm, but its use is limited because it is a technically difficult invasive surgical approach.

Inpatient Versus Outpatient Initiation

Because of the risk of proarrhythmias, including torsades de pointes, most clinicians are understandably wary of initiating antiarrhythmic medications on an outpatient basis. There is limited data to definitively resolve this issue at this time, but the ACC/AHA/ESC Practice Guidelines offer recommendations from the currently available data. Additionally, there are factors that may increase a particular patient's susceptibility to toxicity and, therefore, the decision of where to initiate therapy should be individualized.

Increased toxicity is associated with class IC agents in patients with structural heart disease, depressed LV function, or a widened QRS.

With class Ia or III agents, toxicity is also increased in patients who are female, have structural heart disease or depressed LV function, substantial LVH, renal dysfunction, or electrolyte abnormalities (hypokalemia, hypomagnesemia).

In lone AF, class IC agents (i.e., propafenone, flecainide) can be initiated in outpatients with structurally normal hearts if the patient has tolerated the medication safely as an inpatient in the past. Also remember to administer an AV nodal blocking agent at least 30 minutes prior to the dose.

Although amiodarone prolongs the QT interval, torsades de pointes is uncommon and therefore it is considered safe to administer as an outpatient.

Sotalol is considered safe for outpatient administration in select patients who are in sinus rhythm at the time of initiation and have little or no heart disease, normal electrolytes, and an uncorrected QT interval of less than 460 ms.

Quinidine, procainamide, disopyramide, and dofetilide should not be initiated on an outpatient basis. While initiating antiarrhythmics on outpatients, monitor the EKG weekly with attention to the PR interval, QRS duration, and the QT interval. Also, assess the patient's heart rate and monitor for drug interactions. Reduction of digoxin and warfarin doses is often necessary.

Torsades de Pointes

One of the most concerning adverse events associated with the administration of antiarrhythmics is the development of torsades de pointes. The risk of developing this malignant dysrhythmia while taking a QT-prolonging medication is increased in the setting of hypokalemia, hypomagnesemia, bradycardia, and with higher doses of the medication. The treatment of torsades de pointes is magnesium sulfate 1–2 grams IV over 5–60 minutes.

Chapter 22

Valvular Disease

Introduction

Rheumatic heart disease is the most common cause of valvular disease worldwide; however, in North America and Europe congenital conditions and calcification of the valves as occurs with aging are more commonly encountered. Valvular disorders may also develop as a complication of an acute MI or as a result of trauma or infection.

PAs and NPs often follow patients with valvular heart disease. Appropriate management of these patients requires knowledge of how frequently to monitor with echocardiography, when to consider surgical intervention, and how to medically manage the more common types of valvular disorders.

BACK TO THE BASICS

The heart valves prevent the blood from flowing in the wrong direction. The atrioventricular (AV) valves are located between the atria and the ventricles and prevent the blood from flowing backwards into the atria during systole. The semilunar valves prevent the blood from flowing back into the ventricles during systole.

The chordae tendinea are tendons that link the AV valves to the papillary muscles. The papillary muscles provide tension to prevent the valves from prolapsing into the atria during the high pressure gradient that forces the valves open.

Aortic Stenosis

> **Pearl**
>
> Rheumatic heart disease makes the valves thick and rigid so that they do not open or close completely. As a result, rheumatic heart disease may cause both stenotic and regurgitant valvular disease.

Aortic stenosis (AS) may result from calcific disease, rheumatic heart disease, or a congenital bicuspid valve with superimposed calcification. AS is more common in patients with a congenital bicuspid aortic valve than in patients with normal valve structure. Many of the risk factors for atherosclerosis are also associated with aortic valve sclerosis.

Pathophysiology

Lipid accumulation, inflammation, and subsequent calcification may lead to valvular stenosis. As the stenosis worsens, the resistance to the ejection of blood from the left ventricle into the aorta increases. Essentially, it becomes more and more difficult to push blood through the stenotic valve into the aorta, resulting in the progressive development of a left ventricular outflow tract obstruction. As the volume of blood ejected into the systemic circulation is decreased, the stroke volume, and thus the systolic blood pressure, is reduced. The narrowed valve opening makes it take longer for the blood to be ejected, resulting in a decreased heart rate and a reduction in the amplitude of the pulse.

Additionally, the work demands on the left ventricle are increased as it struggles to force the blood through the narrowed valve opening. This may result in ventricular hypertrophy and eventually heart failure.

Clinical Manifestations

As is often asymptomatic until it increases in severity. It is then associated with a classic triad of dyspnea, dizziness or syncope, and exertional chest pain. The most common symptom of AS is dyspnea on exertion. Arrhythmias may occur once heart failure develops.

On physical examination, you will detect a heart murmur, which is described as a harsh crescendo-decrescendo systolic ejection murmur typically heard best at the base of the heart (2nd right intercostal space) with radiation to the carotid arteries. As AS progresses in severity, the murmur peaks later and later in systole; eventually the S2 may become obliterated by the murmur. You may also hear an S4 at the apex, signifying the decreased compliance of the hypertrophied left ventricle.

The murmur of AS is easiest to hear when the patient is seated, leaning forward. The Valsalva maneuver will decrease the intensity of the murmur because this maneuver decreases the amount of blood ejected into the aorta. Conversely, squatting increases the amount of blood ejected into the aorta and increases the intensity of the murmur. The pulse rises slowly and weakly in patients with AS. This has been described as "pulsus parvus and tardus."

Aortic sclerosis (note sclerosis, not stenosis) is a stiffening of the aortic valve associated with aging; the valve stiffens, but does not obstruct the outflow of blood as in AS. The murmur of aortic sclerosis is also audible at the base of the heart, but peaks earlier in systole, does not radiate to the carotids, and does not obliterate the normal heart sounds.

Diagnosis

If AS is suspected clinically, an echocardiogram is essential to confirm the diagnosis and to assess the severity of the stenosis. The echocardiogram will provide three useful measurements: Doppler peak velocity (aortic jet velocity), mean transvalvular gradient (the pressure gradient from one side of the valve to the other), and aortic valve area. AS is considered to be severe when the valve area is less than 1.0 cm^2, the jet velocity is greater than 4.0 cm^2, and/or the mean gradient exceeds 40 mmHg.

An echocardiogram is recommended in asymptomatic patients annually for severe AS, every 1 to 2 years for moderate AS, and every 3–5 years for mild AS.

Patients with a bicuspid aortic valve are felt to have underlying connective tissue disease that puts them at increased risk of aortic dissection. Therefore, they should have an initial echocardiogram to assess the aortic root diameter and to evaluate the ascending aorta. If dilatation of the aortic root or ascending aorta is present, the patient should be followed with an annual echocardiogram, CT, or MRI to determine the need for surgical repair. Cardiac catheterization is sometimes required to further clarify the severity of valvular dysfunction.

Pearl

When the murmur of AS is louder at the left 2nd right intercostal space rather than the right 2nd intercostal space, an enlarged aortic root or aortic dissection may be present.

Management

Definitive management, which involves replacement of the valve, is essentially reserved for symptomatic patients. Asymptomatic patients can usually be managed conservatively, although surgery may be considered in asymptomatic patients if it is believed that rapid progression may occur or if patients have extremely severe AS.

Surgery is indicated in severe AS if the patient is symptomatic, already undergoing heart surgery for another reason (even patients with moderate AS should have surgical repair if they are already undergoing heart surgery), or has an EF less than 50%. In patients with severe AS who do not meet these criteria, surgery is controversial and an exercise stress test may be considered in order to identify patients who should proceed with surgery. If the patient becomes symptomatic with exercise or develops hypotension, surgery may be considered.

There is no age limit for valve replacement surgery unless comorbid conditions preclude it. Percutaneous balloon valvuloplasty may be considered in younger patients.

> **Pearl**
>
> Because of the increased risk of stressing patients with severe AS, a cardiologist should perform the study rather than a PA, NP, or nurse.

Diuretics and vasodilators such as nitrates should be used cautiously because they may result in profound hypotension. Antibiotic prophylaxis is recommended when patients with AS undergo any procedure that may cause transient bacteremia because these patients are at risk of developing endocarditis.

Aortic Regurgitation

Aortic regurgitation or insufficiency (AI) occurs when an incompetent aortic valve allows blood to flow back into the left ventricle, rather than forward into the aorta, during diastole.

AI may result from an abnormality of the aortic valve itself or dilatation and distortion of the aortic root, which distorts the leaflets, preventing effective closure of the valve. These abnormalities may result from rheumatic fever, endocarditis, trauma, aortic dissection, connective tissue diseases, syphilis, or a congenital bicuspid aortic valve. Although rheumatic disease is the most common cause of AI worldwide, rheumatic disease is now rare in developing countries. For this reason, most chronic cases of AI that are encountered in developing countries are a result of congenital or degenerative causes. Acute AI may be a result of aortic dissection or endocarditis.

Pathophysiology

The incompetent aortic valve allows blood to flow back into the ventricle during diastole, resulting in increased left ventricular end-diastolic pressure (LVEDP).

This causes the left ventricle to increase its stroke volume in an effort to pump a larger quantity of blood during the next contraction. The large stroke volume causes an increased pulse pressure, which translates into systolic hypertension. The increased blood volume leads to ventricular dilatation while the extra pressure and workload of the heart leads to ventricular hypertrophy.

Clinical Manifestations

Chronic AI typically presents insidiously, whereas acute AI usually manifests as severe heart failure with impending cardiogenic shock. Symptoms such as dyspnea or angina do not usually occur until late in the course of the disease.

The characteristic murmur of AI is a decrescendo diastolic murmur. You may also hear an S3 and a low pitch diastolic rumble (Austin Flint murmur) at the apex. The pulse pressure, which is the difference between the systolic and diastolic blood pressure, will be widened.

Palpate the carotid arteries for the classic bounding pulse with a rapid downstroke. This is often called a *water-hammer* or *Corrigan's pulse. Musset's sign,* head bobbing with each heartbeat, may also be evident.

Diagnosis

AI may be suspected on the basis of clinical findings and confirmed by an echocardiography or cardiac catheterization with ascending aortography. The diagnosis of AI is often an incidental finding on an echocardiogram obtained for other reasons.

Management

Asymptomatic patients with normal left ventricular function can be managed conservatively, regardless of the severity of the AI. This entails treating underlying or precipitating causes and echocardiographic monitoring every 6 to 12 months to monitor disease progression.

Antibiotic prophylaxis prior to dental or certain surgical procedures is recommended in all patients with AI despite the low risk of endocarditis. Vasodilators may be considered for patients with moderate or severe AI who are not surgical candidates. Nifedipine may delay the need for AVR in patients with symptomatic AI and normal LV function.

Surgical treatment is reserved for those patients who have developed heart failure symptoms or who have developed LV systolic dysfunction or severely dilated left ventricles or aortic roots. In patients with acute AI and/or hemodynamic compromise, AVR and repair of associated aortic root abnormalities should be performed urgently.

Mitral Stenosis

Mitral stenosis (MS) is predominantly caused by rheumatic fever (more than 99% of cases). Although industrialized countries such as the United States have largely eradicated rheumatic fever and its subsequent valvular disorders, a new wave of patients are immigrating with such disorders.

Pathophysiology

While mitral regurgitation is often seen acutely in patients suffering from rheumatic fever, MS occurs years or decades later. MS is a progressive disorder that involves incomplete opening of the mitral valve, which causes difficulty passing blood from the left atrium into the left ventricle during diastole. This results in an increased volume of blood remaining in the atrium leading to left atrial dilation and increased left atrial pressure due to the increased resistance to pushing blood forward. As the disease progresses, the backup effects the pulmonary circulation and pulmonary hypertension develops.

Clinical Manifestations

Dyspnea, fatigue, and decreased exercise tolerance are the major manifestations. AF and thromboembolism are commonly associated with MS and may be the initial presentation.

The classic MS murmur is a low-pitched diastolic rumbling that begins with an opening snap. It is best heard by placing the bell at the apex during expiration with the patient lying in the left lateral position. You may also notice that the S1 is more pronounced than the S2 at the apex.

> **Pearl**
>
> Use the pneumonic BELL: **B**ell of the stethoscope, **E**xpiration, **L**eft **L**ateral position.

Diagnosis

MS may be suspected on the basis of clinical findings and confirmed by echocardiography.

Management

Medical management is geared toward reducing the hemodynamic impact of obstruction by limiting exercise, adding a beta-blocker or nondihydropyridine CCB, and optimizing volume status with diuretics and salt restriction. Additionally, the patient should receive antibiotic prophylaxis for endocarditis, long-term anticoagulation to address thromboembolic risk, and appropriate management of AF if present.

Percutaneous mitral valve balloon valvotomy (PMBV) is an option for patients with moderate to severe MS that is symptomatic, associated with pulmonary hypertension, or associated with new onset atrial fibrillation. This procedure may also be considered for those patients with moderate to severe symptomatic MS who are not surgical candidates. Mitral valve balloon valvotomy is not indicated in mild MS and should not be performed on patients who have concomitant moderate to severe MR or a left atrial thrombus.

If patients do not qualify for PMBV due to a left atrial thrombus, moderate to severe MR, or a valve structure that is not suitable for PMBV, they may undergo mitral valve repair or replacement as long as they are an acceptable surgical candidate.

Mitral Regurgitation

The most common causes of severe mitral regurgitation (MR) include mitral valve prolapse, ischemia, rheumatic heart disease, and endocarditis while the most common causes of mild MR are systolic dysfunction and ventricular dilatation. Ventricular dilatation stretches the valve apparatus causing ineffective closure. In the elderly, MR is often due to annular calcification. (The mitral valve annulus is a ring around the valve leaflets.)

Acute onset of MR may result from papillary muscle dysfunction after an MI, ruptured chordae tendinae, or by perforation of the valve as in infective endocarditis.

Pathophysiology

Incomplete closure of the mitral valve allows some of the blood to flow back into the left atrium rather than forward into the left ventricle. This added volume in the left atrium causes dilatation and may provoke atrial fibrillation. Additionally, pulmonary pressures may rise.

Clinical Manifestations

Despite the increased workload on the heart, MR is generally well tolerated and many patients remain asymptomatic for years. Patients may initially present with heart failure, atrial fibrillation, or endocarditis, but are more commonly identified by the presence of a murmur or as an incidental finding on an echocardiogram.

On physical examination, the characteristic murmur is a blowing pansystolic murmur best heard at the apex with radiation to the axilla. An S3, a hyperdynamic apical impulse, and a brisk carotid upstroke may be appreciated on exam.

Diagnosis

MR may be suspected on the basis of clinical findings and confirmed by echocardiography.

Management

Careful monitoring of patients with MR is essential in order to arrange valve repair or replacement surgery prior to the development of irreversible left ventricular dysfunction. Surgical repair is preferred over replacement when feasible. Patients with severe MR along with symptoms, left ventricular dysfunction, new-onset atrial fibrillation, or pulmonary hypertension should be considered for surgical repair or replacement.

Because there are inherent risks in undergoing valve surgery, it is not recommended that patients undergo surgery until they become symptomatic or have the comorbidities just listed unless the surgery can be performed at a center with a high success rate such that the benefits of surgery outweigh the risks.

Mitral Valve Prolapse

Mitral valve prolapse (MVP) is characterized by mitral valve leaflets that become enlarged and "floppy" so that they prolapse back into the left atrium during systole.

MVP is often associated with connective tissue disorders and is usually detected in thin, young women with chest wall abnormalities. Although it is usually nonprogressive and benign, it may be associated with supraventricular and ventricular tacharrythmias, such as WPW and Long QT syndrome.

Clinical Manifestations

Most cases of MVP are discovered on routine examination as patients are usually asymptomatic. However, some patients may experience symptoms such as chest pain, dyspnea, fatigue, anxiety, palpitations or light-headedness. The chest pain of MVP may mimic angina, but is prolonged and nonexertional. The pain has been attributed to ischemia resulting from traction of the prolapsing valve leaflets. The anxiety, palpitations, and arrhythmias may result from abnormal autonomic nervous system function that commonly accompanies MVP.

On physical examination, you may hear a midsystolic click followed by a late systolic murmur. It is best heard at the apex and radiates to the left axilla. It is most prominent while standing. Squatting will augment the murmur while Valsalva maneuvers will decrease the murmur.

Diagnosis

MVP may be suspected on the basis of clinical findings and confirmed by echocardiography.

Management

Management of MVP focuses on relieving any symptoms that may be present and ensuring no complications arise. Beta-blockers often provide symptomatic relief in those patients who experience palpitations, mild tachyarrythmias, chest discomfort, or anxiety. Educating patients to avoid stimulants such as OTC cold preparations, caffeine, alcohol, or tobacco may be sufficient to control symptoms.

Infective endocarditis is an uncommon complication and antibiotic prophylaxis is reserved only for those patients with associated MR.

In rare cases, patients with severe valve dysfunction may require valve surgery.

Using Vitamin K for Elevated INRs

Using high doses of vitamin K or administering vitamin K subcutaneously can make it difficult to raise the INR back to therapeutic range when indicated.

If a patient has an INR below 5.0, simply lower the warfarin dose or hold a dose; no vitamin K is needed.

If a patient has an INR between 5.0 and 9.0, first ensure that the patient has no significant bleeding. If not, then you can simply omit one to two doses and monitor the INR more frequently. Be sure to resume warfarin at a lower dose once the INR is back in the therapeutic range. If the patient is at increased risk of bleeding, you can give vitamin K, 1–2.5 mg orally.

If the INR is between 9.0 and 20 with no significant bleeding then hold warfarin and give vitamin K 3–5 mg orally. You can repeat the dose in 24 to 48 hours if not substantially reduced.

If the INR is greater than 20 with serious bleeding, hold warfarin and give vitamin K, 10 mg slow IV infusion. If necessary, you may also give fresh frozen plasma (FFP). Vitamin K can be repeated every 12 hours as needed.

> **Pearl**
>
> It may take 1 to 2 weeks to obtain a therapeutic level of warfarin after administering subcutaneous vitamin K, so try not to use it unnecessarily. (Heparin can be given concomitantly with warfarin if clinically indicated while waiting to achieve therapeutic levels.)

Chapter 23

Rheumatic Fever and Endocarditis

Rheumatic Fever

Rheumatic fever (RF) is one of the sequelae of group A streptococci (GAS) infection. In the United States, RF caused significant morbidity and mortality prior to the advent of antibiotics and prompt treatment of pharyngitis.

Clinical Manifestations and Diagnosis

RF is diagnosed by the presence of two major or one major and two minor Jones criteria and evidence of group A streptococcal infection. Group A strep infection may be confirmed by an elevated antistreptococcal antibody titer, a positive throat culture, or a positive rapid antigen test.

The major Jones criteria include:

- carditis
- polyarthritis
- chorea
- erythema marginatum
- subcutaneous nodules

The minor criteria include:

- fever
- arthralgias
- elevated acute phase reactants
- prolonged PR interval

Carditis may be reflected by a new or significant heart murmur, increasing enlargement of the cardiac silhouette on chest radiography, pericarditis, or congestive heart failure not attributed to another cause. The polyarthritis of RF tends to be migratory and must include signs of inflammation (erythema, tenderness, edema, or increased temperature) or pain associated with limitation of active motion. The chorea associated with RF is called Sydenham's chorea and is an involuntary, irregular, and rapid jerking motion that typically begins in the hands and then becomes more generalized. It may be preceded by inappropriate laughing or crying. Loss of fine motor control, weakness, and hypotonia may also occur. Subcutaneous nodules may be palpated over extensor surfaces of joints, in the occipital region, or the lumbar or thoracic spinous processes. Erythema marginatum is a migratory pink, sharply demarcated rash with a scalloped border and central clearing. It is predominantly located on the trunk, but may also be found on the extremities. It is transient and may be precipitated by heat.

Fever is nonspecific and is, therefore, a minor criterion. Arthralgia may not be used as a minor criterion if polyarthritis has already been used as a major criterion. The presence of leukocytosis and/or the elevation of the erythrocyte sedimentation rate (ESR) or C-reactive protein (CRP) are nonspecific findings associated with inflammation. These and other nonspecific markers for inflammation are considered a minor criterion for RF.

Management and Complications

Prompt treatment of group A strep infections will prevent RF. If a patient develops RF, the goals of treatment are to suppress inflammation, offer symptomatic relief, and eradicate the group A strep.

One of the complications of rheumatic fever is rheumatic heart disease, which damages the heart valves. Mitral stenosis is the most common valvular disorder caused by RF followed by aortic stenosis. All patients who have developed valvular disease as a result of RF require antibiotic prophylaxis to prevent endocarditis.

Bacterial Endocarditis

Endocarditis, infection of the endothelium of the heart, may occur during bacteremia. Transient bacteremia is common during dental, respiratory, urologic, and GI procedures. Endocarditis often affects heart valves, particularly prosthetic or diseased valves. The lesion of endocarditis is called vegetation, which is a mass of the causative microorganism enmeshed in platelets and fibrin.

Rheumatic heart disease is a well-known cause of endocarditis. MVP with MR, congenital heart disease, increased age (due to the increased likelihood of degenerative and calcific valvular disorders), and IV drug use (because of the possibility of introducing microorganisms to the bloodstream during injection) are also associated with increased risk of endocarditis.

The most common organisms associated with endocarditis in native valves are staphylococcus aureus, streptococcus viridans, and enterococci. In patients who develop prosthetic valve endocarditis postoperatively, staphylococcus contamination is likely. If the onset of endocarditis is more than 2 months after surgery, streptococcus viridans is more commonly implicated. In IV drug users, staphylococcus aureus is most commonly the causative agent because it is a normal inhabitant of the skin and is easily introduced through nonsterile injections. Endocarditis that is due to IV drug use commonly affects the right side of the heart.

Acute bacterial endocarditis (ABE) has rapid clinical progression (over 24–48 hours) and is associated with more pathogenic organisms such as staphylococcus aureus. Subacute bacterial endocarditis (SBE) evolves over several weeks to months and is associated with less-virulent organisms such as streptococcus viridans, streptococcus bovis, and HACEK group organisms, which include haemophilus aphrophilus, actinobacillus actinomycetemcomitans, cardiobacterium hominis, eikenella corrodens, and kingella kingae.

Clinical Manifestations and Diagnosis

The patient may have any of the following symptoms: fever, chills, diaphoresis, malaise, cough, arthralgias, myalgias, anorexia/weight loss, back/flank pain, or confusion.

The following may be noted on physical exam:

- Fever
- A heart murmur; present in 85% of patients with endocarditis
- Systemic emboli
- Splenomegaly
- Clubbing of the nails
- Splinter hemorrhages (dark red streaks under the fingernails)
- Osler's nodes (small tender nodules on the finger or toe pads)
- Janeway lesions (small red macules that blanch with pressure and may be present on the palms and soles)
- Roth's spots (Retinal hemorrhages that look like a pale circle surrounded by a red halo)
- Petechiae; often present on the conjunctiva, palate, behind the ears, and on the chest

Order at least three separate blood cultures from three different sites over 24 hours. The ESR, rheumatoid factor, and CRP are usually elevated. A complete blood count, basic metabolic panel, urinalysis, chest radiograph, and EKG are routinely ordered in suspected endocarditis. An echocardiogram is crucial in establishing the diagnosis and sometimes a TEE is needed to obtain a closer look at the affected valve.

The Duke criteria utilize physical exam findings, blood culture results, and echocardiographic findings to diagnose endocarditis. Two major and one minor, one major and three minor, or five minor criteria are required to establish the diagnosis. The criteria are complex and are simplified here for test taking and overview purposes. Please review the guidelines when establishing a definitive diagnosis. The major criteria include:

- Two separate blood cultures positive for organisms typically implicated in endocarditis
- Echocardiographic evidence of endocarditis
- A new regurgitant heart murmur

The minor criteria include:

- A predisposing cardiac condition or IV drug use
- Fever
- Vascular phenomena—major arterial emboli, intracranial hemorrhage, conjunctival hemorrhages, Janeway lesions, septic pulmonary infarcts, or mycotic aneurysm
- Immunologic phenomena—glomerulonephritis, Osler's nodes, Roth's spots, or positive rheumatoid factor
- Microbiological evidence—a positive blood culture that is not adequate to meet major criteria or serologic evidence of a typical organism implicated in endocarditis
- Echocardiographic findings that are consistent with endocarditis but are not adequate to meet major criteria.

Management

An infectious disease consult should be obtained to assist in management and empiric antibiotics should be administered while awaiting consultation and blood culture results. Ampicilllin and gentamycin can be used empirically for SBE and nafcillin should be added to this regimen in ABE.

If the patient is allergic to penicillin, vancomycin may be substituted. The aminoglycosides (gentamycin) are renal toxic (as well as ototoxic) necessitating close monitoring of renal function. Patients who have received 7 or more days of aminoglycoside therapy also require baseline and weekly audiometry testing. Because of their narrow therapeutic window, gentamycin and vancomycin should be monitored with peak and trough blood levels.

Monitor the patient's progress by following the patient's temperature, white blood cell count, and blood cultures. Indications for urgent cardiac surgery include sustained bacteremia while on therapy, refractory heart failure, unstable prosthetic valve, or prosthetic valve obstruction.

Antibiotic prophylaxis is essential in moderate- to high-risk patients when they undergo procedures that may cause transient bacteremia. These include dental, oral, respiratory, GI, or GU procedures including patients undergoing incision and drainage of an abscess or Foley catheter placement if a urinary tract infection is present or suspected.

Patients with the following conditions should be placed on long-term prophylaxis because of the high risk of developing endocarditis:

- Prosthetic heart valve (regardless of type)
- Prior history of endocarditis
- Complex congenital cyanotic heart disease
- Surgically constructed systemic/pulmonary conduits

Additionally, antibiotic prophylaxis is often offered to moderate-risk patients with the following conditions:

- Aortic or mitral regurgitation or stenosis
- Hypertrophic cardiomyopathy
- Mitral valve prolapse, but only if regurgitation is present
- Hemodynamically unstable intracardiac defects
- Intracardiac defects that were repaired within the past 6 months
- Other congenital malformations

Antibiotic prophylaxis is *not* indicated if MR does not accompany MVP. It is not necessary to provide prophylaxis in patients with pacemakers or ICDs or who have CAD or have had CABG. It is also *not* necessary in patients with an isolated secundum atrial septal defect.

For a dental, oral, or upper respiratory procedure, give 2 grams of amoxicillin orally 1 hour prior to the procedure. Clindamycin 600 mg orally, cephalexin 2 g orally, or azithromycin 500 mg orally are a few alternatives in patients who are allergic to penicillin; these alternative medications are also administered 1 hour prior to the procedure.

For GU or GI procedures, give ampicillin 2 grams IV or IM along with gentamycin 1.5 mg/kg IV or IM (maximum 80 mg) 30 minutes prior to the procedure. Then give either amoxicillin 1 gram orally or ampicillin 1 gram IV or IM 6 hours after the initial dose. In patients who are allergic to penicillin, give vancomycin 1 gram IV over 1–2 hours along with gentamycin 1.5 mg/kg IV or IM (maximum 120 mg); both doses should be completed within 30 minutes of beginning the procedure. Low-risk patients can simply be given amoxicillin 2 grams orally 1 hour prior to the procedure or ampicillin 2 grams IM or IV within 30 minutes of starting the procedure.

Complications

Complications of endocarditis include destruction of the valve (which may lead to acute heart failure), neurologic impairment due to emboli, conduction disease, myocardial or brain abscesses, renal impairment (glomerulonephritis, acute renal failure), sepsis, and death.

SECTION IV RESOURCES

Abramowicz, Mark et al. 2004. "Drugs for Cardiac Arrhythmias." *Treatment Guidelines from the Medical Letter* 2 (27): 75–82.

Abramowicz, Mark. 2005. "Drugs for Lipids." *Treatment Guidelines from the Medical Letter* 3(31): 15–22.

American College of Cardiology/American Heart Association Task Force on Practice Guidelines. *ACC/AHA 2005 Guideline Update for the Diagnosis and Management of Chronic Heart Failure in the Adult—Summary Article.* Circulation; 112: 1825–1852.

American College of Cardiology Foundation and American Heart Association. 2004. *ACC/AHA Pocket Guideline: Management of Patients with ST-Elevation Myocardial Infarction.* Antman et al. Circulation. 110 (9) e82. Accessed from http://circ.ahajournals.org/cgi/reprint/110/9/e82. Retrieved June 26, 2006.

American Heart Association. *Heart Disease and Stroke Statistics—2005 Update.* Accessed from www.utdol.com. Retrieved June 26, 2006.

American Heart Association. 1992. "Guidelines for the Diagnosis of Rheumatic Fever. Jones Criteria 1992 Update." *JAMA.* 268: 2069–2073.

Bears, Mark H. 2006. *Merck Manual,* 18th ed. Merck Research Labs.

Bonow, Robert O., Blasé A. Carabello, Kanu Chatterjee, et al. 2006. *ACC/AHA Pocket Guideline Based on the ACC/AHA 2006 Guideline Revision. Management of Patients with Valvular Heart Disease.* Accessed from www.acc.org. Retrieved June 26, 2006.

Braunwald, Eugene, Elliott Antman, John Beasley, et al. 2002. *ACC/AHA Pocket Guideline Update: Management of Patients with Unstable Angina and Non-ST-Elevation Myocardial Infarction. A Report of the American College of Cardiology/American Heart Association Task Force on Practice Guidelines.* Accessed from www.acc.org. Retrieved June 26, 2006.

Bristow, Michael R., Leslie A. Saxon, John Boehmer, Steven Kreuger, et al. 2004. Cardiac-Resynchronization Therapy with or without an Implantable Defibrillator in Advanced Chronic Heart Failure. *The New England Journal of Medicine* 350: 2140–2150.

Burnett, John C. 2005. "Nesiritide: New Hope for Acute Heart Failure Syndromes?" *European Heart Journal Supplements* 7: B25–B30.

Carabello, Blasé A. 2002. "Evaluation and Management of Patients with Aortic Stenosis." *Circulation* 105: 1746–1750.

Carabello, Blasé A and Fred A. Crawford Jr., 1997. "Valvular Heart Disease." *The New England Journal of Medicine* 337(1): 32–41.

Chobanian, A.V., et al. 2003. "The Seventh Report of the Joint National Committee on Prevention, Detection, Evaluation and Treatment of High Blood Pressure." *JAMA* 289(19): 2560–72.

Crawford, Michael, John DiMarco, Walter Paulus, et al. 2004. *Cardiology.* 2nd ed. Mosby. 1071–1105.

Crawford, Peter A. 2004. *The Washington Manual Subspecialty Consult Series: Cardiology Subspecialty Consult.* Lippincott Williams and Wilkins.

DeMaio, Samuel J., Susan H. Kinsella, and Mark E. Silverman. 1989. "Clinical Course and Long-Term Prognosis of Spontaneous Coronary Artery Dissection." *The American Journal of Cardiology* 64(8): 471–474.

DiPiro, Joseph T., Robert L. Talbert, Gary C. Yee. 2005. *Pharmacotherapy: A Pathophysiologic Approach,* 6th ed. McGraw-Hill.

Enriquez-Sarano, Maurice, and A. Jamil Tajik. 2004. "Aortic Regurgitation." *The New England Journal of Medicine* 351:1539–1546.

Exercise Training Meta-Analysis of Trials in Patients with Chronic Heart Failure. 2004. (ExTraMATCH): ExTraMATCH Collaborative. BMJ USA.

Fuster, Valentin, Lars Ryden, et al. 2001. ACC/AHA/ESC Guidelines for the Management of Patients with Atrial Fibrillation: A Report of the American College of Cardiology/American Heart Association Task Force on Practice Guidelines and the European Society of Cardiology Committee for Practice Guidelines and Policy Conferences (Committee to Develop Guidelines for the Management of Patients with Atrial Fibrillation). JACC 38(4).

Gheorghiade, Mihai, and Faiez Zannad. 2005. "Modern Management of Acute Heart Failure Syndromes." *European Society of Cardiology* 7(Supplement B): B3–B7. Accessed from http://eurheartjsupp.oxfordjournals.org. Retrieved July 1, 2006.

Green, G.P., et al. 2004. *The Washington Manual of Medical Therapeutics,* 31st ed. Philadelphia, PA: Lippincott Williams and Wilkins.

Heart Failure Society of America. 2006. "Executive Summary: HFSA 2006 Comprehensive Heart Failure Practice Guideline." *Journal of Cardiac Failure* 12(1): 10–38.

Jones, D.W., and L.J. Appel. 2003. "Measuring Blood Pressure Accurately." *JAMA* 289: 1027–1030.

Mayo Clinic Staff. 2006. *Cholesterol-Lowering Supplements: Another Way to Reduce Cholesterol. Mayo Foundation for Medical Education and Research.* Accessed from www.mayoclinic.com/health/cholesterol-lowering-supplements/CL00013. Retrieved July 1, 2006.

McGinnity, John G., and Mary P. Ettari. 2005. "Non-ST-Segment Elevation Acute Coronary Syndromes." *Advance for Physician Assistants* 13(5–6): 33–39.

National Cholesterol Education Program. 2002. "Third Report of the National Cholesterol Education Program (NCEP) Panel on Detection, Evaluation, and Treatment of High Blood Cholesterol in Adults (Adult Treatment Panel III): Final Report." *Circulation* 106(25): 3143–3421.

Onusko, Edward. 2003. "Diagnosing Secondary Hypertension." *American Family Physician* 67(1): 67–74. Accessed from www.aafp.org/afp/20030101/67.html. Retrieved June 26, 2006.

Otto, Catherine. 2001. "Evaluation and Management of Chronic Mitral Regurgitation." *The New England Journal of Medicine* 345(10): 740–746.

Pasternak, Richard C., Sidney C. Smith, C. Noel Bairey-Merz, et al. 2002. "ACC/AHA/NHLBI Clinical Advisory on the Use and Safety of Statins." *Journal of the American Academy of Cardiology* 40(3): 567–572.

Rose, Megan, and Kim Thrasher. 2002. *Pharmagram for Health Care Professionals.* New Hanover Regional Medical Center, Dept. of Pharmacy.

Porth, C.M. 2005. *Pathophysiology,* 7th ed. Lippincott Williams and Wilkins.

Rutstein, David D., Walter Bauer, Albert Dorfman, Robert E. Gross, et al. 1956. "Jones Criteria (Modified) for Guidance in the Diagnosis of Rheumatic Fever: Report of the Committee on Standards and Criteria for Programs of Care. *Circulation* 13; 617–620. Accessed from http://circ.ahajournals.org. Retrieved December 25, 2006.

Taylor, Eric, Frank Hu, and Gary Curhan. 2006. "Antihypertensive Medications and the Risk of Incident Type 2 Diabetes." *Diabetes Care* 29(5): 1167–1169.

Tierney, L.M., S.J. McPhee, et al. 2005. *Current Medical Diagnosis and Treatment,* 44th ed. Lange.

Up to Date. *Intensity of Lipid Lowering Therapy in Secondary Prevention of Coronary Heart Disease.* Accessed from www.utdol.com. Retrieved June 26, 2006.

Devices

Cardiac devices such as pacemakers, defibrillators, and stents have become commonplace, necessitating that all providers understand some of the basics of these devices.

Chapter 24

Pacemakers

Introduction

Pacemakers are implanted in patients who have a dysfunctional electrical system. The most common reasons for implanting a pacemaker are dysfunction of the SA node (i.e., symptomatic sinus bradycardia or sinus arrest) or high-grade AV block (i.e., type 2 second-degree block or third-degree block).

Pacemakers are usually inserted subcutaneously below the clavicle and leads are inserted via a subclavian vein or cephalic vein cutdown. The procedure is performed under local anesthetic and the patient usually is discharged the following day. When obtaining consent for a pacemaker implantation, be sure that patients are aware of possible complications, which include pneumothorax, cardiac perforation with tamponade, and/or infection. Patients are usually placed on empiric antibiotics to reduce the incidence of infection.

A pacemaker has a pulse generator that produces the pacing impulse and houses the battery. The pulse generator carries the impulse to the heart through catheter wires, which are called leads. There may be one or more leads depending on which chambers of the heart are to be stimulated. The right atrium, right ventricle, and/or left ventricle may all be paced.

A single-chamber pacemaker paces either the right atrium or right ventricle, whereas a dual-chamber pacemaker paces both the right atrium and right ventricle. The advantage of dual chamber pacemakers is that they maintain AV synchrony. A biventricular pacemaker places an additional lead in the coronary venous circulation, which serves to pace the left ventricle. The additional lead provides synchrony between the left and right ventricle, which may improve cardiac output, thereby improving the functional capacity of patients with severe heart failure.

All pacemakers are basically timing devices. They simply count the amount of time it takes from one heartbeat to the next. If it does not detect (sense) a beat in the allotted time, it will deliver a beat (pace) for the patient. If, on the other hand, the pacemaker senses an intrinsic beat, then it will reset its clock and start counting all over again.

A fixed-rate pacemaker paces the heart at the rate that is set by the cardiology provider and this rate does not deviate, regardless of whether the patient's metabolic demands require an increased heart rate. A rate-responsive pacemaker has sensors that detect increased metabolic demand (as with exercise) and adjusts its pacing rate to accommodate the increased demand. This often will improve the patient's quality of life.

For Example

When a VVI pacemaker senses a ventricular signal, it will inhibit a response so that no pacing occurs in the ventricle. If a ventricular signal is not sensed, then the pacemaker will not inhibit its stimulus to pace the ventricle. Thus, a ventricular contraction will ensue.

Pacemakers are described by three to five letters (i.e., DDD, VVI). The first letter indicates which chamber is paced (A = atria, V = ventricle, or D = dual). The second letter indicates which chamber is sensed (A = atria, V = ventricle, D = dual, or O = none). The next letter describes what the pacemaker does when it senses a signal from the heart (I = inhibits a response, T = triggers a response, and D = either response can occur). If a fourth letter is present, it will be an R indicating that the pacemaker has rate-adaptive properties. A fifth letter may denote antitachycardia-pacing abilities.

Electrophysiology PAs and NPs are often responsible for follow-up of pacemaker patients. Close follow-up is essential to ensure the pacemaker parameters are appropriately set, to assess for symptoms, and eventually to determine when the battery is preparing to reach end of life. There is an indicator in the pacemaker that will signal when the battery is near depletion so that a pacemaker generator change-out procedure can be performed.

The process of checking the pacemaker is called interrogation. Pacemakers can also be interrogated over the telephone for the patient's convenience. You will need to know the device's manufacturer so that you can select the proper equipment (programmer) to interrogate the device. The patient should have a wallet card with this information if it is not in the available medical records. Each of the pacemaker manufacturers has a hotline that provides 24-hour technical support including a registry of patients and on-call staff who are available for assistance.

When interrogating a pacemaker, the pacing threshold is assessed. This is the minimum stimulus required to consistently capture the myocardium resulting in depolarization. Optimizing the pacing threshold allows proper function of the pacemaker while preserving battery life.

Sensitivity is the level that a waveform must exceed in order to be sensed by the pacemaker. The sensitivity is another parameter that is assessed during pacemaker interrogation. The correct sensitivity setting ensures that the pacemaker does not visualize baseline artifact, but that it is able to visualize all of the appropriate waveforms, particularly the p waves, which are smaller than the QRS.

Impedance, a measurement of all the forces that oppose the flow of the electrical current, is assessed as well. If the impedance is very low, then lead insulation failure may have occurred. If the impedance is high and the pacing threshold is also high, suspect a lead fracture.

Pacemaker interrogations will also reveal whether any mode switching has occurred. In a dual-chamber pacemaker, the pacemaker can automatically switch to a mode that does not sense in the atrium in the setting of a supraventricular tachycardia. This prevents the pacemaker from sensing the rapid atrial beats, which would have resulted in pacing the ventricle at the fastest rate allowed by the device.

If you intend to work as an electrophysiology provider, you will need more thorough training in the field. The individual pacemaker companies often provide this.

> **Pearl**
>
> Picture the sensitivity as a fence. The higher the fence, the less you will see. In other words, smaller waveforms that may occur with electrical artifact or skeletal muscle movement will not be visible with the sensitivity set high enough to obstruct their view. If the sensitivity is set too high, however, the somewhat taller p waves may also be obscured.

Troubleshooting

Electromagnetic Interference

Pacemakers have built-in filters that prevent interference from most electronic devices such as microwave ovens, motors, and other appliances. However, heavy machinery (i.e., large engines, welding equipment) may affect the pacemaker and should be avoided. A complete list of devices and equipment that may pose a problem is available from **www.guidant.com/patient/living**.

A pacemaker interrogation will reveal any problems that may have occurred in the presence of such equipment or devices.

Pacemaker-Mediated Tachycardia

Pacemaker-mediated tachycardia is a wide-complex tachycardia that may occur in patients who have a pacemaker that is capable of sensing the atrium and pacing the ventricle. Essentially, a PVC may conduct retrograde through the AV node into the atria where it is sensed by the atrial lead. Once this atrial activity is sensed by the pacemaker, it thinks it is supposed to be followed by a ventricular response and paces the ventricle. The pacemaker then becomes part of the reentrant circuit, resulting in tachycardia. To break the tachycardia cycle, simply place a magnet over the device.

Infection

Despite the empiric use of antibiotics during implantation, infection may occur after a pacemaker is implanted. This is usually localized, but is serious. Treatment requires the extraction of the entire system in addition to systemic antibiotics. A new system can be implanted on the opposite side once the infection has resolved.

Twiddler's Syndrome

Twiddler's syndrome occurs when patients intentionally or absentmindedly rotate or manipulate the pacemaker in its pocket. This may result in lead fracture or dislodgement, which will be evident when the device is interrogated. Fixation of the pacemaker along with repair or repositioning of the lead may be required.

Erosion of the Pacemaker

Pacemaker erosion is the protrusion of the device though the chest wall. It has become less common as the devices have gotten smaller, but may occur in patients with thin skin or skin atrophy. If the skin is broken or does not move loosely over the pacemaker, the patient should be managed as if they have an infection.

Extracardiac Stimulation

Pacemakers may inadvertently cause diaphragmatic, phrenic, pacemaker pocket, or pectoral muscle stimulation. This may be a result of improper positioning of the lead, lead insulation failure, or in unipolar pacemakers with high output. Adjusting the output or repair or repositioning of the lead should improve the patient's discomfort.

Pacemaker Syndrome

Patients with pacemaker syndrome may complain of dizziness, syncope, shortness of breath, or pounding/fullness of the head and neck. They may also have hypotension. This is believed to result from lack of AV synchrony, causing less-than-optimum cardiac output. Therefore, AV sequential pacing may improve the patient's symptoms.

Failure to Capture

Capture is the term used to describe the contraction of the myocardium after it has been stimulated by the pacemaker. If the pacemaker provides a stimulus and the myocardium fails to respond with a beat, it is called failure to capture. You can see this on the EKG as a pacemaker spike that does not have a waveform following it. If the atrial lead fails to capture, you will see a pacemaker spike without a p wave following it. If the ventricular lead fails to capture, you will see a pacemaker spike without a QRS following it.

Failure to capture may be a result of a dislodged or incorrectly positioned electrode, lead fracture, insulation break, a fibrosed lead tip, or battery failure. Also, the thresholds may be incorrect. Pacing thresholds may increase in patients with hyperkalemia, myxedema, or with the use of certain antiarrhythmics such as sotalol or propafenone. Pacing thresholds may also increase over time until noncapture occurs.

Failure to Sense

Sensing refers to the pacemaker's ability to detect the heart's own intrinsic beats. If the pacemaker fails to sense, you may see a normal waveform followed by a pacemaker spike (or the spike may even occur in the middle of the waveform) because the pacemaker does not know that the heart conducted its own intrinsic beat and it thinks it has to provide a paced beat.

Failure to sense may be a result of a dislodged electrode, battery failure, or insulation break. Also, the pacemaker thresholds could be set incorrectly so that the pacemaker can't "see" the intrinsic beats. Simply changing the thresholds may correct the problem.

Oversensing occurs when the pacemaker thinks it sees a waveform that is not acutally present or that is artifact or a different waveform. This means the device will not stimulate the myocardium appropriately to produce a beat because it believes a beat is already present.

Chapter 25

Implanted Cardioverter-Defibrillators

Introduction to ICDs

Implanted cardioverter-defibrillators (ICDs) are often implanted to prevent sudden death from ventricular tachyarrhythmias. In addition to administering therapy (shocking patients), all ICDs also function as a pacemaker.

Several types of therapy are employed by defibrillators in an effort to terminate potentially deadly arrhythmias. Antitachycardia pacing provides a low-energy stimulus like that of a normal pacemaker in an effort to terminate tachyaarhythmias without the pain of a shock. Cardioversion is a high-energy electrical shock that is synchronized to the patient's cardiac cycle so that it does not deliver a shock on top of a t-wave, which can induce VT. Another type of high-energy shock is defibrillation, which does not bother to synchronize because it is used on tachyarrhythmias that are so chaotic and disorganized (i.e., VF) that there are no discernible t-waves. Cardioversion and defibrillation shocks are about one million times the energy of a simple pacing pulse.

ICDs try the lower-energy therapies first and resort to the high-energy options in arrhythmias that are more difficult to terminate. This tiered therapy helps to minimize the use of painful shocks unless absolutely necessary. Patients who have experienced a shock from their ICD often describe it as being "kicked in the chest by a horse."

ICDs are indicated in the following circumstances:

- VT or VF cardiac arrest if no reversible cause is identified
- Sustained VT in patients with structural heart disease

- Sustained VT in patients without structural heart disease, but whose VT is not amenable to other treatment approaches (i.e., ablation or antiarrhythmic medications)
- Syncope if hemodynamically significant VT or VF is induced at EP study
- Patients with CAD, prior MI, or LV dysfunction who have nonsustained VT and undergo EP study that induces sustained VT that is not suppressed by class 1 antiarrhythmics
- The MADIT-II study revealed a 31% reduction in mortality in patients with an EF less than 30% who have had an MI at least 1 month ago or CABG at least 3 months ago; hence, an ICD is indicated in these patients as well

ICDs are most effective at preventing sudden death in patients with left ventricular dysfunction. Alternative management (i.e., ablation or pharmacological approaches) are generally preferred to treat VT in structurally normal hearts. Patients who have WPW syndrome, right ventricular outflow tract VT, or other arrhythmias that are amenable to catheter ablation should undergo ablation rather than ICD implantation. Additionally, if the patient has a life expectancy of less than 6 months due to a terminal illness, ICD implantation is not recommended.

ICDs are implanted in much the same way as pacemakers and patients also require close follow-up by ICD specialists who can interrogate the device. PAs and NPs are often employed in this role as well. During an interrogation, battery status can be assessed, lead and device problems can be detected, and a log of arrhythmias and therapies that were delivered can be reviewed.

Pearl

Follow standard ACLS protocols on patients with ICDs if you encounter an arrhythmia. Do not assume that the ICD will handle it. Do not place defibrillator electrodes directly over the ICD. If the patient receives an internal shock while you are making contact with the patient, there is no health risk to you.

If a patient reports that they received a shock from their device, to consider whether the shock was appropriate (VT or VF that met the programmed detection criteria occurred prior to the shock), inappropriate (caused by environmental electrical stimuli or by sinus tachycardia or SVT with a rapid ventricular rate rather than VT or VF), or a phantom shock (the patient perceived a shock that never occurred). Phantom shocks may occur in patients who have had a painful shock previously.

Patients who feel unwell or have received more than one shock in a short period should be evaluated emergently.

Pharmacological therapy should be considered for patients who have received shocks to reduce the odds of having future shocks, but this should be discussed with the patient's electrophysiologist.

In the event of repeated inappropriate shocks, simply place a magnet over the ICD. This disables the ICD, but allows back-up pacing to occur. Once the magnet is removed, the ICD should function normally but you may want to have it interrogated to be certain.

Patients with ICDs should not have an MRI because the strong magnetic fields can interfere with the ICD. However, CT scans, nuclear studies, fluoroscopy, and left heart catheterizations are safe to perform. Patients who are undergoing surgery can have the device turned off during the procedure or have a magnet taped over it.

Caution

Check to see if the device has an advisory or alert because certain alerted devices may have had the magnet function (or other functions) disabled. Simply call the toll-free number of the device's manufacturer when you are not sure.

Pearl

When performing an exercise or dobutamine stress test on a patient with an ICD, you may need to place a magnet over the device to ensure that the patient does not receive a shock if the heart rate rises over the programmed rate for therapy to occur. Simply contact the manufacturer of the device and they will assist you. Alternatively, call the patient's electrophysiologist to find out what the arrhythmia detection rate is set at and discontinue the study if you approach that heart rate.

Chapter 26

Coronary Stents

Introduction

A coronary stent is a wire mesh tube that is permanently placed in a previously narrowed coronary artery. The stent acts as a "scaffolding" to hold the artery open. Stents were initially used in coronary arteries to maintain the patency of the lumen by preventing elastic recoil and tears that were associated with balloon angioplasty.

The problem with early bare-metal stents was the growth of scar tissue inside the lumen of the stent and the increased rate of thrombosis. Essentially, when the metal surface of the stent contacted the blood, a thrombogenic process was naturally initiated. The introduction of dual antiplatelet therapy as well as improvement in technique eventually resulted in restenosis rates superior to ballon angioplasty; restenosis is defined as more than a 50% narrowing at a site of previous intervention. Hence, the use of stents began to escalate such that 90–95% of all percutaneous coronary interventions now involve stent implantation.

The next generation of stents, the drug-eluting stents, were developed with an active coating in an effort to improve restenosis rates. The first drug-eluting stent, the Cypher stent, was produced by coating the stent with a layer of polymer containing sirolimus, which has anti-inflammatory, antiproliferative, and immunosuppressive effects. This was followed by the paclitaxel (Taxus) drug-eluting stent. These stents have reduced the need for reintervention in the treated arteries and are now considered superior to bare-metal stents. However, once the drug has completely eluted from the stent, restenosis may occur, sparking the current controversy regarding the safety of these newer stents.

Thrombosis rates may not have been improved with the newer generation of stents; rather, thrombosis may simply have been delayed. Additionally, hypersensitiviy reactions to the polymer may occur.

To reduce the risk of thrombosis, the society for Cardiovascular Angiography and Intervention now recommends that patients remain on dual antiplatelet therapy with aspirin and clopidogrel for a *minimum* of 3 months (Cypher) or 6 months (Taxus). The society also strongly recommends that patients with drug-eluting stents remain on dual antiplatelet therapy for 12 months or possibly longer. Patients must be advised not to discontinue their antiplatelet therapy within the first year after stenting without consulting their cardiology provider. Additionally, patients must remain on lifelong low-dose aspirin therapy.

SECTION V RESOURCES

Conti, Richard C. 2006. "Drug-Eluting Stents-Safety Concerns." *Clin Cardiol* 29: 479–480.

Crawford, Peter A. 2004. *The Washington Manual Subspecialty Consult Series: Cardiology Subspecialty Consult*. Lippincott Williams and Wilkins.

Gregoratos, Gabriel, et al. 2003. ACC/AHA/NASPE Writing Committee. *ACC/AHA Pocket Guideline Based on the 2002 Guideline Update. Implantation of Cardiac Pacemakers and Antiarrhythmias Devices*. Accessed from www.acc.org. Retrieved December 5, 2006.

Hodgson, John McB., Gregg W. Stone, Michael A. Lincoff, Lloyd Klein, Howard Walpole, Randy Bottner, Bonnie H. Weiner, Martin B. Leon, Ted Feldman, Joseph Babb, and Gregory J. Dehmer. 2007. "Late Stent Thrombosis: Considerations and Practical Advice for the Use of Drug-Eluting Stents: A Report from the Society for Cardiovascular Angiography and Interventions Drug-Eluting Stent Task Force." Published on Behalf of the Society for Cardiovascualr Angiography and Interventions (SCAI) by Wiley-Liss, Inc. Accessed from www. interscience.wiley.com. Retrieved February 20, 2007.

Moses, H. Weston, Joel A. Schneider, Brian D. Miller, and George J. Taylor. *A Practical Guide to Cardiac Pacing*, 3rd ed. Little, Brown, and Company.

Serruys, Patrick W., Michael J.B. Kutryk, and Andrew T.L. Ong. 2006. "Coronary-Artery Stents." *New England Journal of Medicine* 354(5): 483–95.

Stevenson, William G., et al. 2004. "AHA Science Advisory. Clinical Assessment and Management of Patients with Implanted Cardioverter-Defibrillators Presenting to Nonelectrophysiologists." *Circulation* 110: 3866–3869.

Lifestyles

Whether managing patients with cardiovascular disease or proactively preventing future disease, it is essential to address how the patient's lifestyle affects their health. Diet, exercise, and smoking are all critical determinants of cardiovascular risk.

Chapter 27

Heart Healthy Lifestyles

Introduction

Obesity has become a major health problem in many countries including the United States. Poor eating habits, lack of exercise, and stress all contribute to obesity, which contributes to the development of cardiovascular disease. However, even lean patients (those with a BMI less than 25) need to adopt healthy habits to help protect themselves from cardiovascular disease.

In light of the massive amount of false information provided to consumers regarding these issues, it is important that medical providers offer sound advice regarding healthy lifestyle choices. PAs or NPs should aim to inquire about lifestyle choices at each office visit and offer education, motivation, or congratulations as needed.

> **Pearl**
>
> Obese patients are often overwhelmed and disheartened at weight loss efforts because they may have a large amount of weight to lose. It may help to advise them that it only takes a 5% weight loss to achieve important medical benefits. Keeping this in mind, a 300-pound patient can be advised that they only need to drop 15 pounds to reap health benefits. This is very motivating!

Healthy Eating Habits

Hippocrates once said, "Let food be your medicine." While certain foods promote health, it is not always clear which foods are beneficial and which are detrimental. Low-fat diets, which used to be recommended by cardiologists, were subsequently found to aggravate the effect of insulin resistance on blood lipids, effectively worsening one's health. Many physicians are now recommending diets that are more lenient in total fat content, but low in *saturated* fat (less than 10% of total calories). In essence, patients are allowed to eat fatty foods, but they need to distinguish between "good" fat and "bad" fat.

While diet information and misinformation abounds, several foods or diet plans have recently been shown to be heart healthy. The Mediterranean-type diet is a popular diet that has demonstrated significant reduction in cardiovascular morbidity and mortality in multiple studies. The Lyon Diet Heart Study showed a 76% reduction in cardiac mortality and a 70% reduction in total mortality by adopting this type of diet. The Mediterranean diet emphasizes fruits, vegetables, whole grains, beans, nuts, and seeds. Olive oil, which is high in polyunsaturated fat, is the main source of fat. Dairy products, eggs, fish, and poultry are moderately consumed, while red meat and refined sugar is scarce. Wine is consumed moderately with meals.

The following foods have proven health benefits and should be incorporated into a heart healthy diet:

> **Pearl**
>
> It is better to eat a piece of fruit than to drink a glass of juice, because the fiber in the fruit helps slow the absorption of its natural sugars, which prevents sugar spikes and insulin surges.

- Flavonoids: apples, avocadoes, black and green tea, corn, grapes, red wine, string beans, and strawberries
- Isoflavones: tofu, soy nuts, and soy cheese
- Allum/Allicen: garlic, onions, scallions, and shallots
- Fiber: whole grains, fruits, and vegetables
- Eicosapentaenoic acid (EPA) and docosahexaenoic acid (DHA): oils from cold-water fish

Dietary Supplements

Omega-3 Fatty Acids

Many people fear the consumption of fish due to contamination and prefer to take omega-3 fatty acid supplements instead. These have also been proven effective in lowering the risk of heart disease. In the GISSI-preventzione study, patients receiving 1 gram daily of omega-3 fatty acid supplements had a significant 10–15% reduction in the combined primary endpoint of death, nonfatal myocardial infarction, and stroke. Omega-3 fatty acids have been shown to decrease the risk of arrhythmias, lower triglyceride levels, slow the growth of atherosclerotic plaque, and modestly lower blood pressure.

According to the American Heart Association, patients without CHD should eat a variety of fatty fish at least twice a week and incorporate oils and foods rich in alpha-linolenic acid (flaxseed, canola, and soybean oils; flaxseed and walnuts) in their diet. Patients with documented CHD should consume about 1 g of EPA and DHA per day, preferably from fatty fish. Patients who need to lower triglyceride levels should consume 2–4 grams of EPA and DHA per day. Patients consuming high doses of EPA and DHA may have an increased risk of bleeding.

> **Pearl**
>
> Cold-water fish and those that are lower on the food chain have lower mercury levels. Limit exposure to mercury and PCBs by looking for the Ecofish logo on fish that have been tested for these chemicals.

Red Yeast Rice

Red yeast rice contains chemicals that are known to inhibit cholesterol synthesis. One of these chemicals is also known as the drug lovastatin (Mevacor). Studies have shown that red yeast lowers LDL and total cholesterol levels. Adverse reactions may be similar to those of lovastatin and red yeast may also increase the risk of bleeding.

Bottom Line
- Eat more cold-water fish.
- Add onions, garlic, and scallions.
- Drink tea (green and black).
- Eat whole grains and reduce your intake of simple carbohydrates.
- Eat a variety of vegetables and fruit.
- Change to low-fat dairy products.
- Reduce your intake of fatty red meats.
- Choose healthier fats such as olive or canola oils.
- Increase your intake of fiber (beans, whole grains, fruits, and vegetables).

Physical Activity

When starting a patient on an exercise program or increasing their daily activity, it is important to remember safety first. Be sure that patients are familiar with cardiac warning signs. If appropriate, advise patients to have their nitroglycerine accessible and be sure they know how to take it and what to do if it is ineffective. If patients qualify for cardiac rehabilitation, encourage them to enroll.

> **Pearl**
>
> Motivate patients to become more active in small increments in everyday life whenever possible. Simple tasks such as chopping vegetables instead of buying them in presliced packages increases the amount of calories burned.

> **Pearl**
>
> For simplicity, rather than having patients monitor their heart rate, advise them that they should be able to hold a conversation while exercising. If they become too short-winded to converse, then they need to reduce their intensity.

Patients who are extremely sedentary may find it difficult to begin exercising so it is important to stress that any activity is a good start. Gardening burns as many calories as walking and is a more entertaining way for many people to increase their activity levels without becoming bored.

Writing exercise instructions on a prescription pad will underscore the importance of what you are saying. An exercise prescription should include the type of exercise (i.e., resistance exercise to improve strength and aerobic training to improve aerobic capacity), frequency (i.e., 3–5 days/week), and duration (i.e., 20–60 minutes per day).

Patients should aim for a target heart rate of 85%. This can be determined by subtracting the patient's age from the number 220 and then multiplying by 0.85.

Patients will need to start low and go slow. They should increase their activity level as tolerated until they achieve a minimum of 60 minutes of moderate intensity activity (walking briskly) or 30 minutes of vigorous activity (aerobics) daily. This can be divided into two sessions if preferable to the patient. In general, moderate physical activity is that which can be sustained for an hour, whereas vigorous physical activity results in exhaustion after 30 minutes.

The key to maintaining a healthy active lifestyle is to choose activities that are enjoyable. This may mean walking nine holes of a golf game, playing tag with the kids, or working outside in the garden.

Smoking Cessation

Smoking is a known cardiovascular risk factor and cessation is of utmost importance in adapting a heart healthy lifestyle. Ideally, patients should be asked about tobacco habits at every patient contact. If it is determined that the patient is a smoker, advise them of the importance and urgency of smoking cessation and assess their desire to quit.

If the patient expresses a desire to quit, set a quit date and discuss any previous attempts at cessation. Try to discover what led to relapse and what they found helpful during past attempts. Advise the patient to seek support from family, friends, and coworkers, particularly during the critical first few weeks. Encourage the patient to have their spouse or household contacts quit with them or at least have them cease smoking in the house and car.

Discuss pharmacological therapies that may assist their efforts such as OTC nicotine patches, gum, or lozenges. If not contraindicated, provide a prescription for nicotine nasal spray or inhalers, or bupropion SR (Wellbutrin SR).

Provide resources such as the National Quitline at 1-800-QUIT NOW.

Arrange follow-up visits or phone calls for encouragement. If the patient fails, reassure them that relapse is part of the process and encourage them to try again.

Stress Reduction

Although stress is not yet considered an independent risk factor for heart disease, data is beginning to uncover a relationship between stress and the risk of cardiovascular disease. Teaching patients how to better handle stress in their lives is an important part of having a healthy lifestyle. Because providers do not have the time to address stress-reduction techniques in daily practice, I recommend the book *From Stress to Strength: How to Lighten Your Load and Save Your Life* by Robert Eliot, MD.

It is important that patients all have something to look forward to. This may be a once weekly event such as golfing, gardening, or reading an enjoyable book. Ask patients what enjoyable event they have planned in the next 3 months

Pearl

A patient taught me that the best way to initiate a conversation about tobacco cessation is by asking, "How can I help?"

Pearl

I often explain to patients that if oxygen is required on an airplane, parents are instructed to place their own oxygen mask on prior to placing the mask on their child. This illustrates the importance of caring for oneself first in order to be able to continually care for others.

Pearl

When assisting patients in making lifestyle changes, it is helpful to include them in the process. Ask them what they can do to improve their health and then offer practical suggestions to help them achieve their own goals.

and encourage them to plan one if they have not. This could be as exotic as a cruise or as simple as a visit with the grandchildren or a stroll around the botanical gardens.

Patients are often caregivers for loved ones and are under a constant and tremendous strain. It is important to remind these patients of the need for a day of rest.

Bottom Line

The American Heart Association makes the following lifestyle recommendations:

- Achieve and maintain a healthy body weight by balancing caloric intake and physical activity.
- Eat a diet rich in fruits, vegetables, whole grains, and fiber.
- Eat fatty fish at least twice a week.
- Limit saturated fat and trans fat (partially hydrogenated fats).
- Choose lean meats and/or vegetable meat alternatives and fat-free or low-fat dairy products.
- Limit sugar, including beverages that contain sugar.
- Keep alcohol consumption moderate.
- Engage in regular physical activity.
- Avoid tobacco and tobacco products.

SECTION VI RESOURCES

Agency for Healthcare Research and Quality. 2005. *Helping Smokers Quit: A Guide for Nurses.* Accessed from www.ahrq.gov/about/nursing/hlpsmksqt.htm. Retrieved December 27, 2006.

American Gastroenterological Association. 2002. *AGA Guideline: Obesity.* Accessed from www.utdol.com. Retrieved May 11, 2006.

American Heart Association. *Fish and Omega-3 Fatty Acids: AHA Recommendation.* Accessed from www.americanheart.org/presenter.jhtml?identifier=4632. Retrieved January 1, 2007.

American Heart Association. *Stress and Heart Disease: Can Managing Stress Reduce or Prevent Heart Disease?* Accessed from www.americanheart.org/presenter.jhtml?identifier=4750. Retrieved January, 1, 2007.

American Heart Association Nutrition Committee. 2006. *Diet and Lifestyle Recommendations Revision 2006.* Accessed from www.americanheart.org/presenter.jhtml?identifier=3040741. Retrieved January, 1, 2007.

Deen, Darwin. *Exercise: What the Experts Say.* Accessed from www.aecom.yu.edu/family/ugdeenpresents.htm. Retrieved January, 1, 2007.

Eliot, Robert S. 1994. *From Stress to Strength: How to Lighten Your Load and Save Your Life.* Bantam Books.

Gutterson, Connie. 2005. *The Sonoma Diet: Trimmer Waist, Better Health in Just 10 Days.* Meredith Books.

Iestra, J.A., D. Kromhout, Y.T. van der Schouw, et al. 2005. "Effect Size Estimates of Lifestyle and Dietary Changes on All-Cause Mortality in Coronary Artery Disease Patients: A Systematic Review." *Circulation* 112: 924–934.

National Heart, Lung, and Blood Institute Working Group. 2004. *Cardiovascular Consequences of Chronic Stress: Executive Summary.* Accessed from www.nhlbi.nih.gov/meetings/workshops/heart_stress.htm. Retrieved on December 27, 2006.

Natural Standard Research Collaboration. 2006. *Red Yeast Rice* (Monascus Purpureus). Accessed from www.mayoclinic.com/health/red-yeast-rice/NS_patient-redyeast. Retrieved December 29, 2006.

Stone, Neil J. *Lifestyle Interventions: Dietary Therapy, Physical Activity, Weight Control.* Accessed from www.lipidsonline.org. Retrieved April 13, 2006.

Survival Skills

This section is dedicated to clinical year students and new graduates. Becoming a clinician is an enormous responsibility and can be overwhelming initially. I have provided a few hints to help you gracefully ease into your new role.

Chapter 28

Survival Skills

Now that you are a clinician or in your clinical year, you will need some skills to ensure your success. Here are a few to get you started.

Gain Allies

There is nothing worse than having staff members who are unaware of how hard you work or how much knowledge you possess. This may seem insignificant, but remember that these staff members are crucial in making your day better or worse. If your schedule is overbooked, they often strive to ease your load; if a patient is reticent about being asked to see a PA/NP, they will confidently discuss your attributes; when patients complain, they will gently explain that there must be a misunderstanding rather than nodding their head in subtle agreement. When nurses and staff respect you, they help build the trust and respect of others, thereby improving your job satisfaction.

Here are some helpful hints to gain the allies you will need in your day-to-day practice of medicine:

- Nurses, cardiovascular technicians, and medical assistants typically love to learn and understand what you are doing, so teach as you go; this helps them to see your skills and respect your abilities.
- Try to speak positively when you need to correct a staff member. For example you may say, "I have seen it done that way, but I have found that this way works better because . . . ."

- Be calm and collected in emergencies. Nothing will cause you to lose the respect of your staff quicker than panicking in a crisis situation. When a physician is unavailable, all eyes are upon you to help save the day. You need to take a deep breath and keep your wits about you. Call your back-up or code team immediately, remember your ABCs, and keep your panic attack to yourself.
- Acknowledge their efforts. Health care is a naturally stressful job. Schedules are hard to keep, patients call in with a myriad of complaints that are hard to decipher, and physicians are occasionally hard to please. Remember to take the time to thank all those who help you perform your day-to-day tasks and especially thank those who keep spirits high in the office or hospital.
- Advocate for your nurses and staff. Remember that PAs/NPs and physicians earn more than most staff members who are often struggling to support their families. If pharmaceutical representatives want to bring you lunch, encourage them to supply it for the whole office.

Don't Lose Sight of the Forest...

Remember that you entered this profession to help people. Do not let stress or office politics obscure this view. A daily affirmation may help keep you on track. During your commute to work, turn off your cell phone or radio and remind yourself to concentrate on making a difference in someone's life today. Rather than focusing on how long it takes the staff to check in your patients or how a scheduling error dumped a few extra patients onto your schedule, focus on the fact that your patients are scared, hurting, or simply need someone to hear their story. Try to be patient and listen a little longer before redirecting the conversation. However small this may seem, it can profoundly impact the lives of your patients.

Everyone Is Your Teacher

I remember performing my first stress test at the hospital. I had been trained for several months at the office, but always had a physician easily accessible. Now I was essentially on my own. I was nervous and unsure of many things. The nurses and nuclear technicians were extremely knowledgeable and I often sought their advice during those early days. A nurse commented to me many years later that I had been unusually competent when I began working there. I confided in her that I had actually been timid and unsure, but had soaked up all of the staff's knowledge like a sponge.

Everyone Makes Mistakes

During my first few months as a cardiology PA, I was in the ICU searching for a chart in order to perform a consult. I glanced over to where my patient lay and noticed that he appeared blue. I quickly summoned his nurse and asked her to call the critical care physician in charge of his case. I then assessed the patient and determined that he was pulseless and wasn't breathing. A code was called and the nurse and I began CPR.

I was certified but had never actually performed CPR. Although I was exuding confidence, my heart was racing and I was searching for an exit route. As soon as the physician and code team arrived, a kind ICU nurse offered to take my place and continue the chest compressions that I had been delivering. As I gratefully backed away from the bedside, I observed that in my haste I had been administering my compressions over the heart and not directly over the sternum as she was correctly doing.

Needless to say, I was overcome with embarrassment. Every time I saw that critical care physician I kept thinking that he must think I am a total idiot. Imagine a cardiology PA who does not know how to deliver chest compressions correctly!

Several years later, I recounted this story while introducing this physician as a speaker at one of my conferences. When he reached the podium, he announced to the audience that he did not even recall this event, and that I was, in fact, one of the most well-respected PAs in our area.

Remember, we are our own worst critics. I had worried about this physician's opinion of me for many years and he did not even recall the incident. The best way to handle (or avoid) mistakes is to do your best, ask for help, and accept it when you need it; acknowledge and address or rectify your mistakes. Then, let it go.

Take It One Step at a Time

The patient was arriving from an outlying hospital after being resuscitated for a ventricular fibrillation arrest. She was on a respirator and was in critical condition. Her brain function was unknown. Her estimated time of arrival was in 15 minutes and my supervising physician just informed me, the PA with only a few weeks of experience, that the patient was all mine. He would be involved in a catheterization case and would check with me when he was finished.

As I began to have a panic attack right before his eyes, he reassured me by saying that he had complete faith in me and knew I could handle it. Although I appreciated his vote of confidence, I was sure I was incapable of handling this caliber of patient.

Despite my best prayers, the patient eventually arrived. (I was not praying for her death, just to go to another hospital!) She was wheeled in on the gurney and the chart was handed to me. While the paramedics and CCU nurses settled the patient in, I began to review her records. As I read, I began formulating a history of what had happened; I then entered the room and timidly performed a physical exam. As I sat down to complete the history and physical, my supervising physician returned. I presented the case to him and we discussed the plan together.

It was not nearly as bad as I had thought it would be. The trick is that you have to forget about the complexity of the patient and compile your data, using the history and physical format you have learned. Once you gather your data in this organized way, the assessment and plan will flow naturally—and even if it does not, you will be prepared to present the case in a concise format, allowing the physician to guide you in formulating a diagnosis and management plan. So take a deep breath, concentrate on what you have learned, and get to work.

Appendices

Charting Clues

The following charting samples are designed to guide you as you begin to write your own orders. These are only an overview of basic orders and will need to be individualized and updated as the guidelines for treatment change.

Sample Pre-Catheterization Orders

- Have the consent form signed and placed on the front of the chart.

  You must discuss and document the risks, benefits, and alternatives of the procedure. In your note (not orders), write, "R/B/A discussed with patient (and/or family) who understand(s) and agree(s) to proceed."
- Keep NPO post midnight on (date prior to cath), may have clear liquid breakfast if scheduled for late afternoon.
- Valium 5 mg po, benadryl 25 mg po, and IV D5/ NS @ 100cc/hr on call to cath lab. (If the patient has CHF, reduce rate to 50 or KVO as clinically indicated.)
- D/C glucophage for 48 hours before (if possible) and after catheterization.
- D/C lovenox before midnight the night before. (If ordering admission labs, choose heparin over lovenox if there will not be enough time for two doses of lovenox prior to midnight before cath.)
- Serum B-HCG

  Order if the patient is a woman of child-bearing age because of the radiation used for fluoroscopy during the procedure.

- IV dye prophylaxis

  If the patient has a history of IV dye allergy or an allergy to shellfish, order IV dye prophylaxis. Each cardiologist will have his or her own preferred regimen, but here is one example (give all three medications):

  Prednisone 60 mg po at 6 PM and midnight the evening before cath and 6 AM on the day of cath, hydrocortisone 100 mg IV on call to cath lab, and benadryl 50 mg IV on call to cath lab.
- Renal Protection

  If the patient is at risk for contrast-induced nephropathy (i.e., a diabetic with a creatinine greater than 2.0 prior to the procedure), administer IV fluids and consider:

  Mucomist 600 mg BID given on the day before and day of the cath. (Give with orange juice because it tastes really bad.) Weigh the risks and benefits of cath with regard to renal risks.

Sample Status/Post Stent Orders

- D/c lovenox
- EC-ASA 325 mg po qd
- Plavix 75 mg po QD
- F/u 1, 3, and 6 months (some physicians prefer 1, 6, and 12 months)
- No heavy lifting or bending for 48 hours (for groin protection)
- No prolonged sitting (i.e., long car rides) for 1 week
- No tub baths or swimming for 5 days

Sample Pre-Pacemaker Orders

- Have the consent form signed and placed on the front of the chart.

  You must discuss and document the risks, benefits, and alternatives of the procedure. In your note (not orders), write, "R/B/A discussed with patient (and/or family) who understand(s) and agree(s) to proceed."

  The Risks include: 1/500 Bleeding, infection, pneumothorax or < 1/1000 lead dislodgement, perforation, or cardiac tamponade.
- Keep NPO
- IV ancef 1 gm on call (Use vancomycin if elevated creatinine or allergic to cephalosporins.)
- Place IV in left arm
- Void on call

Sample Orders: Suspected or Known AMI

- Admit to CCU
- Dx: Acute MI
- Condition: Critical (or guarded)
- Activity: BR with BRP (This means bed rest with bathroom privileges; remove bathroom privileges if clinically indicated.)
- VS q routine (typically q 30 mins × 4; q 60 mins × 2; if stable then q 4–6 hrs through 24 hours and then q 6 hours thereafter)
- Heart healthy diet with no added salt; diabetics will also require a diabetic-type diet (these have various names, so see what it is called at your hospital)
- IV fluids (as clinically indicated) i.e., "IV: KVO with 5% D/W"
- O2 @ 2 L/min via nasal cannula (more if indicated)
- ECG q 8 hours × 3
- Portable CXR on admission
- Daily weights and intake/output
- Labs:
  Serum markers of myocardial infarction q 8 hours × 3 (CK, CK-MB, troponin, myoglobin)
  Electrolytes (BMP or chem 7) QD × 2–3 days
  H and H
  Lipids (Order a random level within first day of admission, because lipid panels are altered by an AMI, so your results will be inaccurate if you wait for a fasting level.)
  PT/PTT if on heparin, coumadin, or if precath
- Meds:
  Colace 100 mg po qd prn constipation
  ASA 325 mg po qd
  Ativan 0.5 mg po q 6 hours prn anxiety
  Morphine 5 mg IV q 30 mins prn severe pain (Be sure that a strict drug protocol is in place.)
  Plavix
  B-blocker
  Statin
  ACEI
- Precath orders if indicated

Elements of a Discharge Summary

- Date of admission
- Date of discharge
- Reason for admission
- Pertinent history and physical
- Hospital course: summarize the treatment, progress, any complications, consults, or procedures
- Discharge disposition: where they are going next (i.e., home, assisted living, rehab)
- Discharge condition: i.e., good, stable, fair, guarded, critical
- Discharge medications
- Discharge instructions: activity, diet, symptoms to monitor
- Follow-up: next appointment, who to call in an emergency; consider enrolling in a CHF telephonic program or Lincare's Heart Steps program in CHF patients

RESOURCES

Alpert, Joseph S., and Gary S. Francis. 2000. *Handbook of Coronary Care*, 6th ed. Philadelphia, PA: Lippincott Williams and Wilkins, 31–36.

Suggested Resources

Pharmacology

The Medical Letter is a nonprofit publication with no known vested interests that presents evidence-based pharmacology in a very practical and easy-to-read manner.

Up-to-Date Information

Up to Date Online accessed at **www.utdol.com** is an excellent resource for information on any medical topic or disease state. This requires a subscription; ask your doctor or administrator for access to this great resource.

EKG Interpretation

Rapid Interpretation of the EKG by Dale Dubin is a great book that was recommended by my supervising physician when I began working as a PA in cardiology. I loved it because you can read it in one or two nights and there are "cheat sheets" to stuff in your labcoat until you become proficient at reading an EKG.

Cardiology CME Conference

I may be biased about this one because I am the founder of the company, CME Opportunities, LLC. However, this is the only conference that I am aware of that is designed by a cardiology PA specifically for cardiology PAs and NPs. Check out **www.cme-opportunities.com** for more information.

NMR Lipoprofile

Call the customer service center (1-877-547-6837) for more information about ordering this expanded lipoprotein analysis as discussed in Chapter 18.

Mediteranean-Type Diet Book

The Sonoma Diet by Connie Guttersen, RD, PHD, is an excellent reference for patients in need of a heart-healthy diet.

Pharmaceutical Assistance for Patients

Instruct patients to view the following Web sites: **www.rxassist.org** or **www.needymeds.com** if they are having trouble affording their medications.

Information About Alternative Medications and Supplements (as Well as Traditional Medications)

Access this Mayo Clinic resource at:
www.mayoclinic.com/health/search/drugSearch.

Electromagnetic Interference in Patients with Pacemakers or ICDs

For a list of appliances and equipment to avoid in patients with electronic devices, go to **www.guidant.com/patient/living**.

Smoking Cessation

Provide the patient with the toll-free number for the national quitline: 1-800-QUIT NOW.

Free Education Program for Patients with Heart Failure

The HeartSteps program provided by Lincare is provided in the patient's home at no charge. This is an excellent resource for parents. They will learn about their disease, foods they should avoid, how to weigh themselves, and more. Call your local Lincare representative or check out **www.lincare.com**.

Index

---

page numbers followed by "t" or "f" denote tables or figures respectively

CPSIA information can be obtained
at www.ICGtesting.com
Printed in the USA
BVOW00s0458101116

467453BV00002B/4/P